LIFETIME FITNESS

Edward L. Fox

Professor of Physical Education
Director, Laboratory of Work Physiology
School of Health, Physical Education and Recreation
The Ohio State University
Columbus, Ohio

Illustrated by Nancy Allison Close

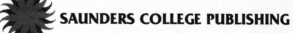

SAUNDERS COLLEGE PUBLISHING

Philadelphia   New York   Chicago
San Francisco   Montreal   Toronto
London   Sydney   Tokyo   Mexico City
Rio de Janeiro   Madrid

Address orders to:
383 Madison Avenue
New York, NY 10017

Address editorial correspondence to:
West Washington Square
Philadelphia, PA 19105

Text Typeface: Press Roman
Compositor: TechType Graphics
Acquisitions Editor: John Butler
Project Editor: Sally Kusch
Copyeditor: Mary Agre
Managing Editor and Art Director: Richard L. Moore
Design Assistant: Virginia A. Bollard
Text Design: Phoenix Studio
Cover Design: Richard L. Moore
Text Artwork: Nancy Allison Close
Production Manager: Tim Frelick
Assistant Production Manager: Maureen Read

Cover credit: Artwork drawn by Tom Mallon

Library of Congress Cataloging in Publication Data

Fox, Edward L.
　　Lifetime fitness.

　　(Saunders physical activities series)
　　Bibliography: p.
　　Includes index.
　　1. Exercise—Physiological aspects.　　2. Physical fitness.
　　3. Health.

　　I. Title.　II. Series.
QP301.F68　1982　　　613.7　　　82-60504

ISBN 0-03-059738-2

LIFETIME FITNESS (SPAS)　　　　　　　　　　　　　　ISBN 0-03-059738-2

345　090　98765432

CBS COLLEGE PUBLISHING
Saunders College Publishing
Holt, Rinehart and Winston
The Dryden Press

*Dedicated to my family for their
love and support in all I do*

PREFACE

More today than ever before, Americans are fitness-conscious. Also more today than ever before, scientific information is continuing to mount in favor of a definite positive relationship between fitness and health — the higher your fitness level, the better your health status.

Keeping fit, however, is not easy. It requires constant dedication and sincere commitment. It involves not just occasionally setting aside a little time for exercise, but an entire change in lifestyle. There are no quick and easy remedies, although all of the gimmicks available and testimonials would make you believe just the opposite.

This book contains basic but scientifically sound information regarding how to increase your fitness level. It was written for everyone willing to learn how to improve and maintain his or her fitness. For the young reader, now is the time to get in the habit of exercising your way to a lifetime of fitness and good health. For the older reader, remember, it's never too late to start!

I would like to thank John Butler of Saunders College Publishing for his patience and his usual good help and guidance during the preparation of this book. I would also like to thank Dr. Norman Kaluhiokalani for his valuable contributions concerning muscular strength and weight resistance programs. Last, but certainly not least, I would like to thank my wife, Ann, for her endless encouragement and assistance during the writing of the manuscript.

EDWARD L. FOX
Columbus, Ohio

CONTENTS

1☐Introduction to Lifetime Fitness

There is little doubt that regular physical activity is a significant factor in reducing the severity of cardiovascular and other diseases among the peoples of the world, particularly in the United States. Of all deaths in the United States, more than half are due to cardiovascular diseases. As shown in Figure 1–1, cardiovascular diseases and their incidence in the United States include: (1) heart attack: 34%; (2) stroke: 11%; (3) hypertensive diseases: 3%; and (4) other: 6%.

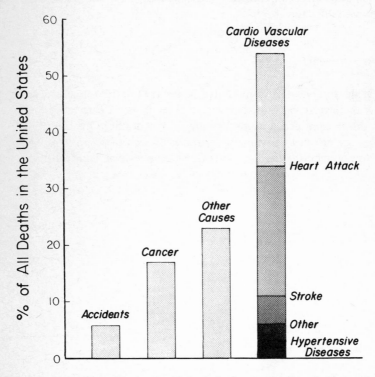

Figure 1–1. Of all deaths in the United States, more than half are due to cardiovascular disease.

Another major health problem in the United States is obesity (overfatness). As with cardiovascular diseases, more than 50 percent of all adults are afflicted with obesity. The incidence of cardiovascular disease is statistically and physiologically related to obesity. For example, the obese individual has a mortality rate from cardiovascular disease that is 2½ times greater than the individual with an average or below average body composition or weight. Since the major cause of obesity is physical inactivity, this means that regular exercise training can significantly reduce both the problems of obesity and cardiovascular diseases.

With these thoughts in mind, the major purposes of this chapter are to discuss the causes and risk factors of cardiovascular diseases and to define fitness and its components.

CAUSES AND RISK FACTORS OF CARDIOVASCULAR DISEASES

To start our discussion of exercise and health, a brief overview of some of the causes and risk factors associated with cardiovascular diseases will be presented.

As mentioned previously, the most common types of cardiovascular diseases are: (1) heart attack or coronary heart diseases; (2) stroke or apoplexy; and (3) hypertensive diseases.

Causes of Heart Attack

Of the total deaths in the United States due to cardiovascular diseases, heart attack or coronary heart disease accounts for about 65 percent. This means that heart attack alone accounts for 35 percent of all deaths in the United States!

The major cause of coronary heart disease is *atherosclerosis,* a slow, progressive disease involving the narrowing of the arteries that supply the heart muscle with blood. These arteries are referred to as the coronary arteries. This narrowing is in turn caused by fatty substances (e.g., calcium and other cellular sluffings) being deposited on the inside walls of the arteries. Besides the narrowing effect, the arteries so afflicted sometimes become stiff or hardened, thus the term "hardening of the arteries." As shown in Figure 1–2, the narrowing is progressive

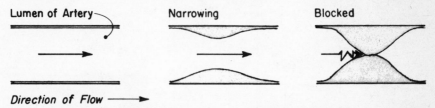

Figure 1–2. The narrowing of the lumen of an artery by atherosclerosis is progressive. In an advanced stage, the blood flow through the artery can be completely blocked.

and, in advanced stages, the blood flow through the artery can be completely stopped. When this occurs, that part of the heart muscle dies that was supplied with blood by that artery, and a heart attack is said to have occurred. The severity of the heart attack is determined by the exact location of the block within the artery. For example, as shown in Figure 1–3, if the block is toward the end of the artery, then the heart attack may not be too severe since the amount of heart tissue involved would be minimal. However, if the block is more toward the beginning of the artery, the amount of tissue involved would be large and the heart attack severe.

Because atherosclerosis is a relatively slow-developing disease, it is generally thought of as an "old age" disease. However, this is not necessarily true. For example, autopsies on American soldiers killed in the Korean and Vietnam wars have revealed moderately advanced stages of atherosclerosis in a majority of these young men. The beginning stages of atherosclerosis have also been found in children less than 5 years of age, and 62 percent of the children between the ages of 7 and 12 years have been found to have at least one coronary heart disease risk factor.

Risk Factors Associated with Heart Attack

It was stated earlier in this chapter that regular physical activity is a significant factor in reducing the severity of heart attacks. Thus, one risk factor

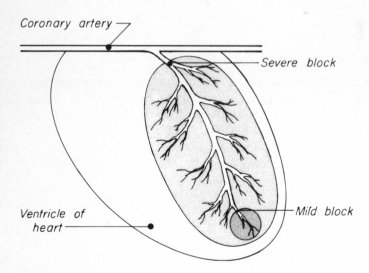

Figure 1–3. A heart attack occurs when the blood flow through a coronary artery is blocked. If the block is toward the end of the artery, the heart attack may not be too severe since the amount of heart tissue involved would be minimal. However, if the block is more toward the beginning of the artery, the amount of tissue involved would be large and the heart attack severe.

that has been identified with heart attacks is physical inactivity or sedentary living. How to properly prescribe an exercise program for the purpose of reducing the risk of heart attack will be discussed in detail later in this book. Right now, some of the other known risk factors associated with heart attack will be discussed.

Age

Generally, the older you are, the greater is your risk for heart attack. For example, between the ages of 25 and 34 years, the death rate due to heart attack is about 10 in every 100,000 white men; at age 55 to 64 years, this rate increases one hundredfold to nearly 1,000 deaths in every 100,000 men.

Heredity

Heredity appears to play some role in the risk of heart attack. For example, people who suffer heart attack, particularly at an early age, have a family history of early age heart attacks. By the same token, those who do not have heart attacks generally belong to families where heart attacks rarely strike.

The exact way in which heredity plays a role in heart attack is not known at this time. Rather than being genetically linked, there is the possibility that family life styles, including eating habits and physical exercise patterns, are more important in developing the tendency toward heart attack. In other words, parents who rarely exercise on a regular basis tend to raise children who also rarely exercise. Obesity is another good example; obese parents frequently raise obese children.

Obesity

As mentioned previously, the risk of heart attack increases as the proportion of body fat increases. People who are considered 20 percent or more overfat have a mortality rate from cardiovascular disease that is 2½ times greater than people with average or below average body weight. Remember, the most common cause of obesity itself is lack of exercise. Weight loss through exercise and dieting is an effective remedy for obesity. These topics will be discussed in more detail in Chapter 6.

Cigarette smoking

The more cigarettes smoked per day and the longer one smokes, the greater the risk of coronary heart disease and lung cancer. As shown in Figure 1-4, a person who smokes more than one pack a day has over twice the risk of heart attack compared with the nonsmoker. Although the link between lung cancer and smoking is quite well known by the general public, its link to coronary heart disease is not.

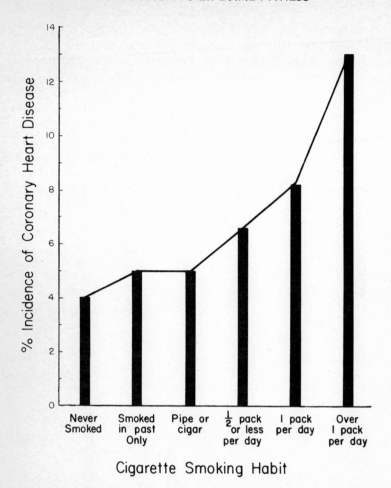

Figure 1–4. Percent incidence of coronary heart disease in relation to cigar-ette smoking. A more than one-pack-a-day smoker has over twice the risk of heart attack compared with the nonsmoker.

Exercise

Many studies have been conducted in hopes of finding conclusive evidence that increased physical activity decreases the risk of coronary heart disease. Most of these studies, however, have failed to do so. Instead, the majority of studies have only been able to *infer* that exercise and coronary heart disease are related. Nevertheless, so many studies have arrived at this same conclusion that it is strongly accepted as fact.

One of the first studies to infer that exercise and coronary heart disease are related was conducted in 1953 in England with groups of bus drivers and bus conductors. The results showed that the incidence of heart disease in the seden-tary bus drivers was twice that of the more active bus conductors. While the drivers sat most of their working day, the conductors walked up and down the double-decker buses. Since this study nearly 30 years ago, many similar studies using different groups of subjects have come to the same conclusion: *the risk of heart attack is less the more physically active you are.*

Blood cholesterol levels

The American diet is typically very rich in foods containing large amounts of animal fats and cholesterol. Animal fats, in turn, are rich in saturated fats. Both cholesterol and these fats make up a large part of the atherosclerotic deposits on the inner lining of the arteries. In this way, high blood levels of cholesterol and triglycerides (saturated fats) are related to a high incidence of coronary heart disease. Such a relationship is shown in Figure 1–5. Note that the incidence of

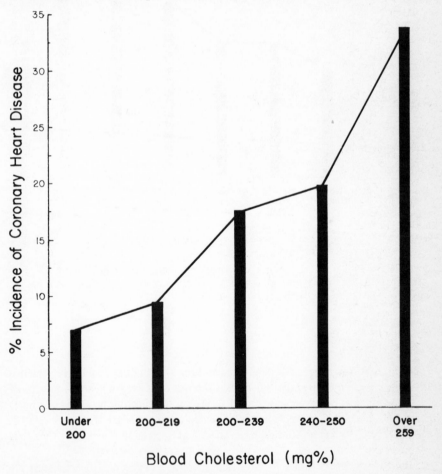

Figure 1–5. Percent incidence of coronary heart disease in relation to blood cholesterol levels. Note that the incidence of coronary heart disease of a person with a blood cholesterol of over 259 mg % is nearly 5 times that of a person with a blood cholesterol of under 200 mg %.

coronary heart disease in a person with a blood cholesterol of over 259* is nearly five times that of a person with a blood cholesterol of under 200. The blood levels of cholesterol and saturated fats can be reduced by avoiding foods rich in these substances and by substituting vegetable fats (unsaturated fats) for animal fats. Regular physical activity has also been shown to reduce blood cholesterol levels.

Blood pressure (hypertension)

High blood pressure or hypertension is another risk factor associated with coronary heart disease. As shown in Figure 1–6, an individual with a systolic blood pressure* of over 150 millimeters of mercury (mm Hg) has over twice the risk of coronary heart disease than does someone with a pressure below 120 mm Hg. It is estimated that 15 percent of the entire United States population

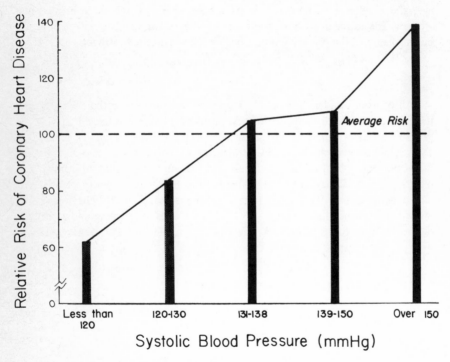

Figure 1–6. Relative risk of coronary heart disease in relation to systolic blood pressure. An individual with a systolic blood pressure of over 150 mm Hg has over twice the risk of coronary heart disease than does someone with a pressure below 120 mm Hg.

---

*The unit of measure most commonly used with blood cholesterol measurements is milligrams per 100 milliliters of blood (abbreviated mg percent). One milligram = 1/1000 of a gram = 0.000035 ounces.

*Systolic blood pressure is the pressure obtained when the blood in the heart is ejected or emptied into the arteries.

suffers from hypertension. For adults in the United States, about 20 percent of white men and women have hypertension and about 30 percent of black men and women are hypertensive. Of these, the majority are classified as "essential," meaning that no known cause (and therefore, no known cure) can be identified as causing the hypertension. Another astonishing fact is that essential hypertension in young children and young adults is on the increase in the United States. Once again, regular physical activity has been shown to be effective in reducing blood pressure to nearly normal values.

Sex

The incidence of coronary heart disease is greater in young men than in young women. For example, the death rate of white men between the ages of 35 and 44 years is six times that for white women of the same age. However, with older age, the incidence of coronary heart disease is about the same in men and women. The lower death rate due to heart disease among young women is probably related to the production of a female hormone called estrogen.

Stress

All of us are under "pressure" or stress at one time or another. While this in itself is not necessarily bad, the biggest problem is how we manage it. Two basic types of behavior in response to stress have been identified: *Type A* and *Type B*. Type A behavior is characterized by high levels of aggression, competition, and drive. For example, Type A individuals always seem to be "racing the clock," no matter what it is they are doing. This type of behavior has been scientifically linked with increased risk of coronary heart disease. Type B behavior, on the other hand, is just the opposite of Type A, that is, easy going and seemingly never in a hurry to beat the clock. The risk of coronary heart disease is much less with Type B behavior than with Type A.

The three big risk factors

Of all the previously mentioned risk factors, the three most important are: (1) cigarette smoking; (2) high blood pressure; and (3) high blood levels of cholesterol. The danger of a heart attack with none or a combination of these risk factors is shown in Figure 1–7. If all three primary risk factors are present, the danger of a heart attack is five times that when none is present!

What is Your Coronary Heart Disease Risk?

The Michigan Heart Association has published a gamelike test called Risko that may be used to estimate your chances of suffering a heart attack.

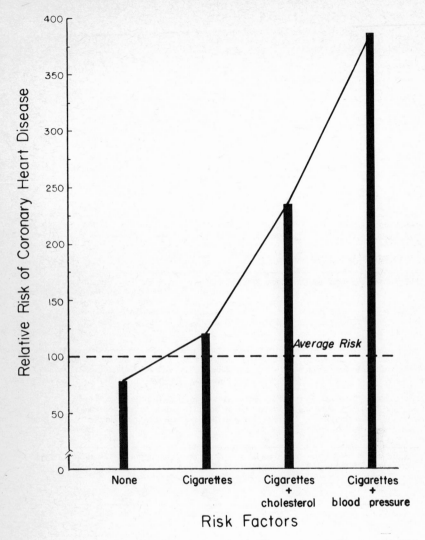

Figure 1-7. Relative risk of coronary heart disease in relation to the "big three" risk factors. If all three primary risk factors are present, the danger of a heart attack is 5 times that when none are present.

The game is played using Table 1-1 by marking squares that — from left to right — represent an increase in your **risk factors**. These are medical conditions and habits associated with an increased danger of heart attack. Not all risk factors are measurable enough to be included in this game.

TABLE 1-1   Cardiac Risk Index

1 Age	10 to 20	21 to 30	31 to 40	41 to 50	51 to 60	61 to 70
	1	**2**	**3**	**4**	**6**	**8**
2 Heredity	No known history of	1 relative over 60 with cardiovascular disease	2 relatives over 60 with cardiovascular disease	1 relative under 60 with cardiovascular disease	2 relatives under 60 with cardiovascular disease	3 relatives under 60 with cardiovascular disease
	1	**2**	**3**	**4**	**6**	**8**
3 Weight	More than 5 lbs below standard weight	−5 to +5 lbs standard weight	6–20 lbs overweight	21–35 lbs overweight	36–50 lbs overweight	51–65 lbs overweight
	0	**1**	**2**	**3**	**5**	**7**
4 Tobacco smoking	Nonuser	Cigar and/or pipe	10 cigarettes or less a day	20 cigarettes a day	30 cigarettes a day	40 cigarettes or more a day
	0	**1**	**2**	**4**	**6**	**10**
5 Exercise	Intensive occupational and recreational exertion	Moderate occupational and recreational exertion	Sedentary work and intense recreational exertion	Sedentary work and moderate recreational exertion	Sedentary work and light recreational exertion	Complete lack of all exercise
	1	**2**	**3**	**5**	**6**	**8**
6 Cholesterol or % fat in diet	Cholesterol below 180 mg%	Cholesterol 181–205 mg%	Cholesterol 206–230 mg%	Cholesterol 231–255 mg%	Cholesterol 256–280 mg%	Cholesterol 281–330 mg%
	No animal or solid fats in diet	10% animal or solid fat in diet	20% animal or solid fat in diet	30% animal or solid fat in diet	40% animal or solid fat in diet	50% animal or solid fat in diet
	1	**2**	**3**	**4**	**5**	**7**
7 Blood pressure	100 upper reading	120 upper reading	140 upper reading	160 upper reading	180 upper reading	200 or over upper reading
	1	**2**	**3**	**4**	**6**	**8**
8 Sex	Female under 40	Female 40–50	Female over 50	Male	Stocky male	Bald stocky male
	1	**2**	**3**	**5**	**6**	**7**

Total score_____

Rules

Study each risk factor and its row. Find the box applicable to you and circle the number in it. For example, if your age is 37, circle the number in the box labeled 31–40. After checking out all the rows, add the circled numbers. This total — your score — is an estimate of your risk.

If you score:

6 – 11 ...Risk well below average
12 – 17 ...Risk below average
18 – 24 ...Risk generally average
25 – 31 ...Risk moderate
32 – 40 ...Risk at a dangerous level
41 – 62 ...Danger urgent. See your doctor now

Heredity. Count parents, grandparents, brothers, and sisters who have had heart attack and/or stroke.

Tobacco smoking. If you inhale deeply and smoke a cigarette way down, add one to your classification. Do not subtract because you think you do not inhale or smoke only a half inch on a cigarette.

Exercise. Lower your score one point if you exercise regularly and frequently.

Cholesterol or saturated fat intake level. A cholesterol blood level determination is best. If you can't get one from your doctor, estimate honestly the percentage of solid fats you eat. These are usually of animal origin — lard, cream, butter, and beef and lamb fat. If you eat much of this, your cholesterol level probably will be high. The United States average, 40 percent, is too high for good health.

Blood pressure. If you have no recent reading but have passed an insurance or industrial examination, chances are you have an upper reading of 140 or less.

Sex. This line takes into account the fact that men have between six and ten times more heart attacks than women of child-bearing age.

Causes of Stroke and Hypertensive Diseases

According to the American Heart Association, a stroke occurs when there is interference with the blood supply to the brain. In order to function, brain cells must have a continuous and ample supply of oxygen-rich blood, which if completely stopped, causes the cells to die. One of the frequent causes of stroke is the blocking of one of the arteries that supplies blood to a section of the brain by a clot that forms inside the artery. This is a condition called *cerebral* (brain) *thrombosis*. A clot is not likely to occur in a healthy artery. However, in arteries damaged by atherosclerosis, clots are apt to form around the deposits formed on the inner wall of the artery. Thus, a major cause of stroke is atherosclerosis.

Stroke also occurs when an atherosclerotic artery in the brain bursts, flooding the surrounding tissue with blood. This is called a *cerebral hemorrhage*. Cells nourished by the artery are deprived of blood and cannot function. The accumulation of blood from the burst artery soon forms a clot. By displacing or destroying brain tissue, it may interfere with brain function, causing physical disability.

A cerebral hemorrhage is more likely to occur when a person suffers from a combination of atherosclerosis and high blood pressure. For example, the risk of stroke if you are a 45-year-old man, smoke cigarettes, have a high blood cholesterol level and high blood pressure is over 10 times that of a man of the same age with none of these risk factors. Hemorrhage of an artery in the brain may also be caused by a head injury or by a burst *aneurysm.* Aneurysms are blood-filled pouches that balloon out from a weak spot in the artery wall and are often associated with high blood pressure. Aneurysms do not always cause trouble, but when one bursts in the brain the result is a stroke.

The result of a stroke is usually *hemiparesis* or paralysis of one side of the body. It also may result in *aphasia,* the loss of the power of expression or understanding communications or in the loss of memory. The effects may be slight or severe, temporary or permanent, depending on which brain cells have been damaged and how widespread the damage is. Effects also depend on how well the body can repair its system of blood supply or how rapidly other areas of the brain tissue can take over the work of the damaged cells.

Prevention of stroke through modification of risk factors is particularly important since injured brain cells cannot be replaced. Regular exercise can reduce the risk of stroke because of its effects on blood cholesterol and blood pressure.

DEFINITIONS AND COMPONENTS OF FITNESS

Now that we know that regular physical activity can lead to a reduction of the risk of cardiovascular and other diseases, we need to concentrate on the end result of regular physical activity, that is, an increase in our level of fitness. In order to do this, we need to know how fitness is defined and to clearly identify its components.

Definition of Fitness

Fitness means different things to different people, and therefore its meaning can sometimes be complex and confusing. However, for our purposes, the meaning of fitness will be simple and clear: fitness implies a *physiological* or *functional capacity* that allows for an improved *quality of life.* Two important concepts in our definition of fitness are "physiological or functional capacity" and "quality of life." The meaning of both of these needs to be expanded in order to fully appreciate the concept of fitness.

What is a physiological or functional capacity?

Capacity is usually expressed as a volume, for instance, the capacity of a glass is 8 ounces. A physiological or functional capacity also refers to volume. For example, the physiological or functional capacity of the heart and lungs (circulatory and respiratory systems) refers to the volume of blood and thus oxygen that can be delivered to the skeletal muscles during exercise. The greater this capacity, the greater the ability of the muscles to contract or work for long periods of time. In terms of fitness, this kind of capacity is related to what is referred to as endurance fitness, aerobic fitness, cardiorespiratory fitness, or cardiovascular fitness. By definition then, endurance or cardiorespiratory fitness refers to the capacity or ability of the heart-lung system to deliver blood and thus oxygen to the working muscles during prolonged physical exercise. The greater this capacity, the greater the endurance fitness level.

The skeletal muscles also have physiological or functional capacities. One of these capacities is related to how much force a muscle or muscle group can exert during contraction. This capacity is more commonly referred to as strength. Another physiological or functional capacity of skeletal muscle is concerned with the length of time a muscle can continue to exert force without fatiguing. This is known as local muscular endurance. It should be emphasized here that muscular endurance differs from cardiorespiratory endurance in that the latter depends more heavily on the heart-lung system for delivering blood and oxygen to the muscles.

Another capacity of the muscles involves the joints. The range of motion that is possible about the joint over which a muscle spans is called joint flexibility or more simply flexibility. In terms of fitness then, muscular fitness is concerned with muscular strength, muscular endurance, and joint flexibility.

Other kinds of fitness do not always relate to specific physiological or functional capacities such as cardiorespiratory fitness and muscular fitness. Instead, the fitness is more general and involves several physiological capacities or functions. A good example of this kind of fitness is nutritional fitness. By definition, nutritional fitness is concerned with proper selection of foods with regard to their nutrient and caloric values as well as proper eating habits. Nutrition affects all bodily functions and therefore involves most physiological systems. For example, good nutrition promotes optimal body growth and development and prevents a whole host of diseases. In other words, good nutritional habits or nutritional fitness, along with good exercise habits, help ward off the overfat syndrome in which the body accumulates excessive amounts of fat.

Mental and emotional fitness and motor fitness are other examples of fitness that involve several of the body's physiological systems. Mental and emotional fitness is concerned with coping with tension and other stresses that are encountered on a daily basis. One of the ways to relieve built-up tension is through physical exercise. Actually, some physicians have found that for many of their emotionally stressed patients, regular participation in an exercise program is a better prescription than any kind of chemical medication. In other words, the "good" feeling experienced by many joggers and other regular exercisers may very well be simply a result of temporary relief from mental and emotional stress.

Motor fitness is concerned with abilities related to physical skills such as endurance, power, strength, agility, flexibility, balance, and coordination. This kind of fitness is similar to that possessed by an all-around athlete.

The components of fitness. Hopefully, most of you have already noticed that the above discussion not only included the definition of a physiological or functional capacity, but also a list of the various components of fitness. However, in case some of you missed the latter point, let's review what these components are.

Component One: Cardiorespiratory or Endurance Fitness.　This is defined as the capacity or ability of the heart-lung system to deliver blood and thus oxygen to the working muscles during prolonged physical exercise.

Component Two: Muscular Fitness.　This kind of fitness has three subcomponents: (a) *muscular strength,* which is defined as the force a muscle or muscle group can exert during contraction; (b) *muscular endurance,* defined as the length of time a muscle or muscle group can continue to exert force without fatiguing; and (c) *joint flexibility,* which is the range of motion possible about a joint over which a muscle spans.

Component Three: Nutritional Fitness. Nutritional *fitness* is concerned with proper selection of foods with regard to their nutrient and caloric values as well as proper eating habits.

Component Four: Mental and Emotional Fitness.　These are concerned with coping with tension and stresses encountered on a daily basis.

Component Five: Motor Fitness.　This kind of fitness is concerned with abilities related to physical skills such as endurance, power, strength, agility, flexibility, balance, and coordination.

These fitness components are reviewed in Table 1–2. It should be pointed out at this time that this book will be concerned only with the first three components of fitness, namely, cardiorespiratory fitness, muscular fitness, and nutritional fitness.

TABLE 1–2　Components of Fitness

FITNESS COMPONENT	DEFINITION
Endurance fitness	Capacity of the heart–lung system to deliver blood and thus oxygen to the working muscles during prolonged physical exercise
Muscular fitness	Muscular strength is the capacity of a muscle or muscle group to develop force during contraction. Muscular endurance is the capacity of a muscle or muscle group to continue to contract without fatiguing. Flexibility is the range of motion possible about a joint over which a muscle spans
Nutritional fitness	The proper selection of foods with regard to their nutrient and caloric values as well as proper eating habits
Mental or emotional fitness	Coping with tensions and stresses encountered on a daily basis
Motor fitness	The abilities related to physical skills such as endurance, power, strength, agility, flexibility, balance, and coordination

What does quality of life mean?

One last concept that needs to be cleared up is the meaning of the phrase "quality of life." You will recall that quality of life is an important phrase in our overall definition of fitness. What generally is meant by quality of life is an overall positive feeling and enthusiasm for life. Fatigue and exhaustion from routine day-to-day activities prevent us from increasing the quality of our lives. On the other hand, an increased level of fitness enables us to perform these routine tasks without undue fatigue and thereby allows us to participate in the activities we most enjoy.

2 □ The Physiology of Fitness

Although fitness was defined and the various components of fitness were discussed in the last chapter, we still need to briefly review some of the basic physiological systems of the body. Three systems will be reviewed: (1) the energy producing systems; (2) the heart-lung or cardiovascular and respiratory system; and (3) the muscular system.

METABOLISM – THE ENERGY-PRODUCING SYSTEM

Various physical activities involve specific demands for energy. For example, sprinting, jumping, and throwing are high power output activities requiring large bursts of energy over short periods of time. Marathon running, distance swimming, and cross-country skiing, on the other hand, are mostly low power output activities requiring small but sustained energy production. Still other activities demand a blend between bursts of energy and sustained energy production. The energy producing system of the body (more simply called metabolism) is responsible for supplying the energy demanded by these various activities.

Metabolism – What is It?

The term *metabolism* refers to the various series of chemical reactions involved in energy production that take place within the human body. Some of these reactions can only occur in the presence of the oxygen we breathe while others can occur in the absence of oxygen. Those reactions that require the presence of oxygen are called *aerobic* (aerobic = with oxygen); those not requiring oxygen are called *anaerobic* (anaerobic = without oxygen). Basically then, there are two ways whereby energy can be produced within the body: (1) through aerobic metabolism; and (2) through anaerobic metabolism.

16

The Immediate Energy Source — ATP

Contrary to popular belief, the energy released from the food we eat is not directly used by the cells for work. Instead, a chemical compound called *adenosine triphosphate,* or, more simply, *ATP,* is the immediately usable form of chemical energy for the body's various functions, including muscular contraction. ATP is stored in most cells, particularly muscle cells. Other forms of chemical energy, such as that available from the foods we eat, must be transferred into the ATP form before they can be utilized by the muscle cells.

The chemical structure of ATP is complicated, but four our purposes it may be simplified as shown in Figure 2–1A. As shown in the figure, ATP consists of a large complex of molecules called adenosine and three simpler components called phosphate groups. The last two phosphate groups represent "high energy bonds." In other words, they store a high level of potential chemical energy. When the terminal phosphate bond is chemically broken, as shown in Figure 2–1B, energy is released, enabling the cell to perform work. The kind of work performed by the cell depends on the cell type. For example, mechanical work (contraction) is performed by muscle cells, nerve conduction by nerve cells, secretion by secretory cells, and so on. All "biological" work performed by any cell requires the immediate energy derived from the breakdown of ATP.

The transfer of food energy into the ATP form occurs, as mentioned before, through two series of metabolic reactions referred to as either aerobic, when sufficient oxygen is present, and/or anaerobic, when sufficient oxygen is not available.

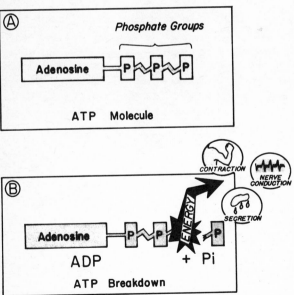

Figure 2–1. (A) ATP consists of a large molecule called adenosine and three simpler components called phosphate groups. (B) The energy released from the breakdown of ATP is used to perform biological work.

Supplying ATP through Anaerobic Metabolism. The ATP energy needed to perform activities that require large bursts of energy over short periods of time, such as sprinting, is supplied primarily through anaerobic metabolism. The reason for this is that these activities are performed so rapidly that not enough oxygen can be delivered by the heart-lung system to the working muscles. Thus, the ATP energy must be supplied in the absence of sufficient oxygen.

The major component involved in anaerobic metabolism is one of the *foodstuffs, carbohydrates* (sugars). This foodstuff in either its simplest form as glucose or in its storage form as glycogen* is chemically broken down inside the cell to a substance called *lactic acid.* During its breakdown, energy is released and some of it is captured as ATP energy (see Figure 2–2). However, the lactic acid that is formed causes temporary muscular fatigue when it accumulates in the blood and muscles. Therefore, reliance on anaerobic metabolism soon causes muscular fatigue. This is one of the reasons why we fatigue so rapidly when we perform activities such as sprinting. Specifically designed training programs like those practiced by sprinters can improve the capacity for anaerobic metabolism.

Supplying ATP through Aerobic Metabolism. The ATP energy needed to perform activities that require a sustained energy production, such as long dis-

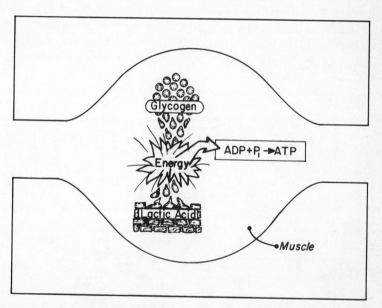

Figure 2–2. The major component involved in anaerobic metabolism is the foodstuff carbohydrates (glycogen as shown here). It is chemically broken down inside the cell to lactic acid. During its breakdown, energy is released, and some of it is captured as ATP energy.

---

*Glycogen is the storage form of glucose and is stored in both the liver and skeletal muscles.

tance running or swimming, is supplied primarily through aerobic metabolism. During the performance of these kinds of activities, enough time is available so that the heart-lung system can deliver sufficient amounts of oxygen to the working muscles.

As with anaerobic metabolism, the foodstuff carbohydrate (glucose and glycogen) is a major ingredient in the series of aerobic chemical reactions. But, unlike anaerobic metabolism, two other foodstuffs, *fat* and *protein* can also enter into the aerobic reactions. However, during exercise, carbohydrates and fats, but generally not proteins, are the important metabolic foodstuffs.

Carbohydrates or fats are chemically broken down in the presence of oxygen inside the cell to carbon dioxide and water. During their breakdown, energy is released and some of it is captured as ATP energy (see Figure 2–3). As just mentioned, these reactions occur inside the muscle cell, but are confined to specialized compartments within the cell called *mitochondria*. Mitochondria (singular = mitochondrion) are slipper-shaped cell bodies often referred to as the "power-houses" of the cell because they are the seat of the aerobic reactions that lead to ATP production. As you might guess, muscle cells are rich with mitochondria.

The by-products of the aerobic breakdown of carbohydrates and fats, which are carbon dioxide and water, do not cause muscular fatigue. In fact, the carbon dioxide that is produced diffuses freely from the muscle cell into the blood and is carried to the lungs where it is exhaled. The water that is formed is useful within the cell itself, since the largest constituent of the cell is, in fact, water.

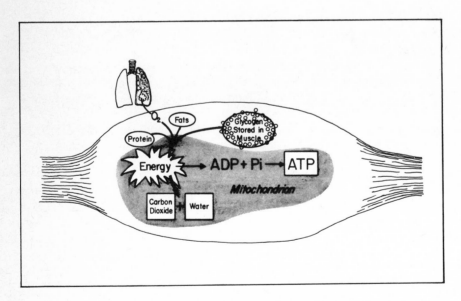

Figure 2–3. The oxygen, or aerobic, system. The aerobic breakdown of carbohydrates, fats, and even proteins provides energy for ATP resynthesis. Since abundant ATP can be manufactured without yielding fatiguing by-products, the aerobic system is most suited for endurance activities.

Since no fatiguing by-products are formed during aerobic metabolism, it is easy to see that this system of providing ATP energy is particularly well suited for endurance-type activities (e.g., long-distance running and swimming). In addition, since oxygen is a requirement, circulation and respiration are important support systems for aerobic metabolism. Herein lies one of the connections between cardiorespiratory or endurance fitness and coronary heart disease. As we will learn in the next chapter, specific exercise training programs can be constructed to increase the capacity for aerobic metabolism.

A summary of the characteristics of the energy producing system is given in Table 2–1.

Energy Production and Nutritional Fitness

It was mentioned in the first chapter that nutritional fitness involves many physiological systems. The link between the metabolic system and nutrition is obvious. For example, as has just been discussed, the foodstuffs (carbohydrates, fats, and proteins), when broken down, provide the energy that is transferred into the ATP form. Also, when a given amount of oxygen is taken in to help break down a given amount of foodstuff, a given number of calories is said to be expended. More about nutrition, energy expenditure, and calories will be discussed in a later chapter.

THE CIRCULATORY AND RESPIRATORY SYSTEMS – THE OXYGEN TRANSPORT SYSTEM

As was emphasized before, the circulatory and respiratory systems, sometimes referred to as the cardiorespiratory system, are responsible for delivering oxygen to the working muscles during prolonged exercise. The oxygen, of course, is used for aerobic metabolism. In this light, another name, the *oxygen transport system*, seems appropriate. A brief description of the functional aspects of this system is as follows: First, as shown in Figure 2–4, the respiratory system provides a means whereby air is moved into and out of the lungs.

TABLE 2–1   Summary of the Characteristics of the Energy-Producing System

CHARACTERISTIC	ENERGY SYSTEM	
	Aerobic	Anaerobic
Oxygen required	yes	no
Foodstuff used	Carbohydrates (glucose, glycogen), fats, proteins	Carbohydrates
Fatiguing by-products	none	Lactic acid
Activities used for	Endurance or long-duration activities	Sprint or high-intensity, short-duration activities

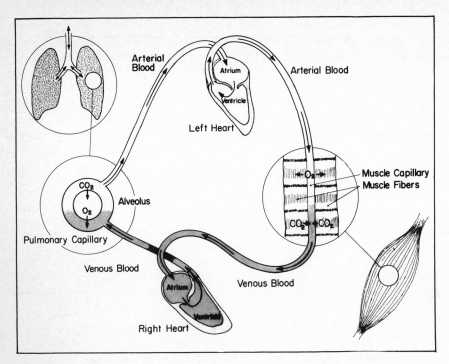

Figure 2–4. The cardiorespiratory system. The respiratory and circulatory systems work intimately together in meeting, under all conditions, the gaseous exchange and transport requirements of the cells.

This rhythmic to-and-fro movement of air is called *pulmonary ventilation.* Next, the oxygen brought in from the outside environment through pulmonary ventilation is made available to the blood by a vast network of small blood vessels called *capillaries* that surround the 600 million or so tiny closed air sacs or *alveoli* found deep within the lungs. The blood contained within the capillaries is *venous blood,* which is relatively low in oxygen and high in carbon dioxide content. At the *alveolar-capillary membrane* oxygen moves by a physical process called *diffusion* from the air in the alveoli to the blood in the capillaries, whereas carbon dioxide diffuses in the opposite direction. Thus, the venous blood brought to the alveoli of the lungs via the right side of the heart returns to the left side of the heart as *arterial blood,* which is high in oxygen and low in carbon dioxide. The alveolar-capillary membranes, then, represent a functional union between the respiratory and circulatory systems.

The next important job, which is the transporting of arterial blood to the body tissues (and ultimately the carrying of venous blood away from the body tissues), is carried out by the left side of the heart and its associated blood vessels. It should be remembered here that the heart represents two muscular pumps, each with its own circuit of blood vessels. As has already been pointed out, the right side of the heart and its blood vessels are primarily responsible for transporting venous blood to and arterial blood from the alveoli of the lungs.

This is called the *pulmonary circuit* or *pulmonary circulation*. Maintaining an adequate flow of arterial blood to and venous blood from the body tissues, on the other hand, is the primary function of the left side of the heart and blood vessels. This is called the *systemic circuit* or *systemic circulation*.

Referring again to Figure 2–4, arterial blood in the pulmonary circuit is returned to the left side of the heart, which then pumps it to all of the body tissues — for instance, in our example, to the skeletal muscles. At this level, another vast network of capillaries is found. Skeletal muscles are richly supplied with capillary beds that come into close contact with the individual muscle fibers. It is at these *tissue-capillary membranes* that a second exchange of gases occurs. This time, oxygen diffuses from the blood in the capillaries to the cells of the tissues, and carbon dioxide diffuses in the opposite direction. The exchange of gases at the tissue-capillary membranes converts arterial blood to venous blood. The venous blood is then returned to the right side of the heart, where the entire process of exchange and transportation of gases is repeated over and over again.

Finally, as has just been discussed, the oxygen delivered via the cardiorespiratory system is utilized by the muscle cells for purposes of supplying energy in the form of ATP.

Pulmonary Ventilation, Blood Flow, and Heart Rate during Exercise

When the demand for oxygen increases, such as during exercise, the stress placed on the oxygen transport system increases tremendously. For example, the amount of air taken in from the environment under resting conditions is only about 6 to 8 liters every minute (a liter = 1.057 quarts). However, during maximal exercise this increases to 125 to 150 liters per minute!

Other cardiorespiratory responses are also exaggerated during exercise. For instance, the amount of blood pumped by the heart in one minute, called the *cardiac output,* increases from 5 or 6 liters per minute at rest to as high as 30 liters per minute during maximal exercise (see Figure 2–5). Actually, in highly trained distance runners, the value during maximal exercise may be as high as 40 liters per minute, which is over 42 quarts of blood! This tremendous increase in blood flow is a result of two basic changes in the response of the heart.

The first of these changes is an increase in the amount of blood pumped by the heart muscle with each beat or stroke. This is referred to as the *stroke volume.* During rest, it may be only 70 milliliters (0.7 liter), whereas during maximal exercise it increases to 110 to 120 milliliters per stroke.

The second change in the response of the heart that causes a great increase in blood flow is an increase in the number of times the heart beats per minute. This is referred to as the *heart rate* and probably is familiar to most of you. For instance, the heart rate, or actually the *pulse rate,* may be counted by placing your first two fingers (index and middle fingers) on the skin over a large artery.

Cardiac Output (Liters/min.)

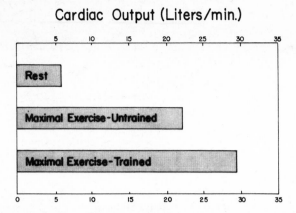

Figure 2–5. The amount of blood pumped by the heart in one minute, the cardiac output, increases from 5 or 6 liters per minute at rest to as high as 30 liters per minute during maximal exercise. Endurance training increases the maximal attainable cardiac output.

(We will later learn how to take advantage of this information in prescribing exercise programs.) The heart rate, at rest, is normally somewhere between 65 and 85 beats per minute. During maximal exercise, however, the heart rate can increase to as high as 200 beats per minute in young, healthy individuals.

The responses of the stroke volume and heart rate to exercise are shown in Figure 2–6.

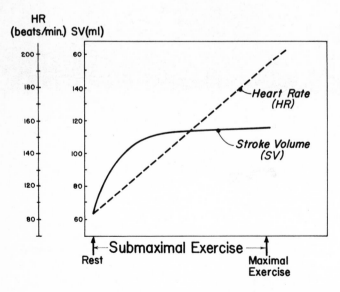

Figure 2–6. To meet the tremendous increase in blood flow required during exercise, both the stroke volume and the heart rate increase during exercise.

THE MUSCULAR SYSTEM

There are basically three kinds of muscle in the human body: (1) *heart muscle;* (2) *smooth muscle;* and (3) *skeletal muscle.* We already mentioned the heart earlier in this chapter. Smooth muscles are found in the walls of the blood vessels, in the gastrointestinal tract, and in other internal organs. Although the smooth muscles are obviously important, we will not need to discuss them further. Skeletal muscles, on the other hand, move the bony skeleton (hence their name) and, therefore, are capable of producing motion. These muscles will be the major focus of our discussion of the muscular system.

Structure and Function of Skeletal Muscles

As shown in Figure 2–7, the connective tissues* of skeletal muscles are of three kinds: the *endomysium,* which surrounds the fibers or cells; the *perimysium,* which surrounds the bundles; and the *epimysium* that encases the entire

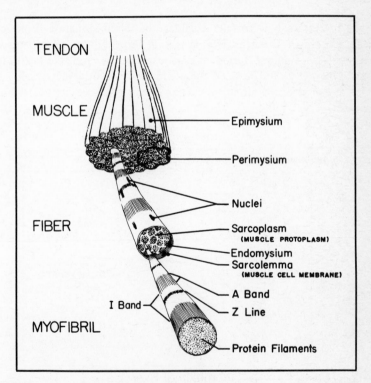

Figure 2–7. The structural and functional subunits of skeletal muscle.

---

*Connective tissue binds together and is the support of the various structures of the body.

muscle. The cell membrane of the muscle fiber is called the *sarcolemma.* The connective tissues become continuous with the connective tissues of the tendons; the latter connect the skeletal muscles to the bony skeleton.

Each muscle fiber or cell contains hundreds of threadlike protein strands called *myofibrils,* within which the contractile unit is housed (see Figure 2–8). The light and dark striations of the myofibrils are called the *I* and *A bands,* respectively. The bands contain two protein filaments, *actin* and *myosin.* Myosin filaments have tiny protein projections called *cross bridges* that extend toward the actin filaments.

Muscular contraction, according to the *sliding filament theory,* results when the actin filaments are pulled over the myosin filaments, thus producing tension and shortening of the muscle (Figure 2–9). Both shortening and tension development are dependent upon (1) the breakdown of ATP for energy; (2) the presence of calcium; and (3) the coupling of myosin to actin (formation of actomyosin).

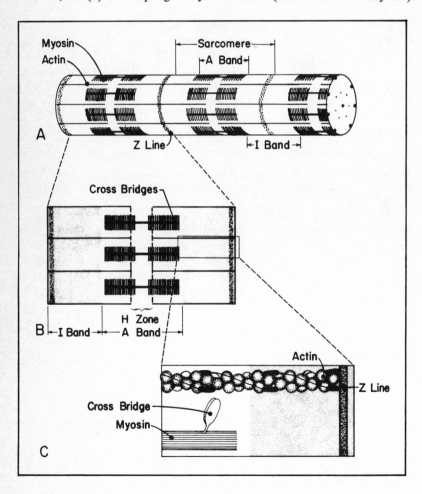

Figure 2–8. Detailed structure of the myofibril.

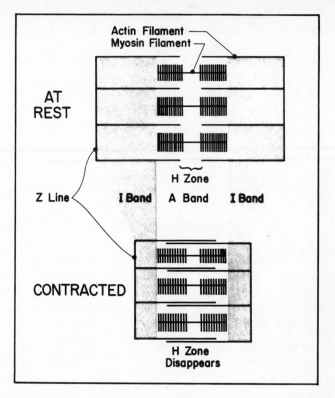

Figure 2–9. The sliding filament theory of muscular contraction. When a muscle contracts isotonically, the actin filaments slide over the myosin filaments.

Muscles are richly supplied with blood vessels. On the average, three to four capillaries surround each fiber in sedentary men and women, whereas five to seven surround each fiber in male and female athletes.

Muscles contain both *motor* and *sensory nerves.* Motor nerves originate in the *central nervous system* (brain and spinal cord) and when stimulated cause the muscles to contract. The termination of a motor nerve on a muscle fiber is known as the *motor end plate* or *neuromuscular junction.* Sensory nerves convey information concerning pain and orientation of the parts of the body from the muscle to the central nervous system.

Most motor nerves have many branches and thus, in entering a muscle, supply many muscle fibers. However, a given muscle fiber is supplied by only one motor nerve. A motor nerve plus all the muscle fibers it supplies is called a *motor unit* (see Figure 2–10). The motor unit is the basic functional unit of skeletal muscle. When the motor nerve of a motor unit is stimulated, all the muscle fibers within that unit contract together. If there are many muscle fibers in the unit, the contraction will be strong. However, if there are only a few muscle fibers within a unit, the contraction will be weak. The response of the muscle can thus be graded depending upon the size and number of motor units stimulated. Such an arrangement allows for fine, delicate movements as well as for gross, large-scale movements.

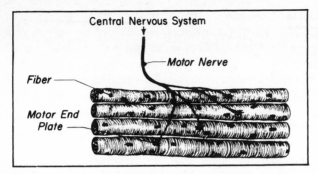

Figure 2–10. Motor unit of skeletal muscle. A single motor nerve from the central nervous system is shown supplying several muscle fibers through the motor endplates (neuromuscular junctions).

Although all skeletal muscle motor units function in the same general manner described above, the muscle fibers within a given motor unit may be either *fast twitch* or *slow twitch fibers*, but not both. Fast twitch fibers (or motor units) have a high capacity for anaerobic metabolism and a low capacity for aerobic metabolism. On the other hand, slow twitch fibers have a high capacity for aerobic metabolism and a low capacity for anaerobic metabolism. During exercise, the slow twitch fibers are mainly used for endurance activities whereas the fast twitch fibers are mostly used for sprintlike activities.

Types of muscular contraction

There are four basic types of muscular contraction. All of them are used to various extent during different kinds of physical activities.

1. Isotonic Contraction. In this type of contraction, the muscle shortens as it develops tension. It is the most familiar type of contraction, being used in all lifting activities, including most weight-training programs (see Chapter 4 for more on weight-training programs). Other names for this type of contraction are *dynamic contraction* and *concentric contraction.*

2. Isometric Contraction. The word isometric means same (iso) length (metric). During an isometric contraction, the muscle develops tension but does not change length. This is also a familiar type of contraction. Holding a weight at arm's length or attempting to lift an immovable object are both examples of isometric contractions. Isometric contractions also occur during sports performance, such as in wrestling. Another name for isometric contraction is *static contraction.*

3. Eccentric Contraction. This is just the opposite of an isotonic or concentric contraction. During eccentric contraction, the muscle lengthens as it develops tension. A good example of this type of contraction is during the performance of "negative work," such as when you are lowering a weight or resisting a movement or gravity. During downhill running and walking down stairs, the muscles are eccentrically contracting. It is easy to see that this type of contraction is also frequently used during the performance of various activities as well as in many sports performances.

4. Isokinetic Contraction. This is a rather "new" type of contraction, at least as applied to sports performance. It is defined as a maximal contraction at constant speed (iso = same, kinetic = motion) over the full range of movement. Such contractions are common during sports performances, a good example being the arm stroke during freestyle swimming. Isokinetic and isotonic contractions are both concentric contractions, the main difference being that during an isokinetic contraction the speed of the contraction or movement is constant.

To perform a controlled isokinetic contraction, special equipment is required.* Basically, the equipment contains a speed governor so that the speed of movement is constant no matter how much tension is produced in the contracting muscles. Thus, if one attempts to make the movement as "fast" as possible, the tension generated by the muscles will be maximal throughout the full range of motion, but the speed of movement will be constant. The movement speed on many isokinetic devices can be pre-set, and can vary between 0 and 200 degrees of motion per second. Many movement speeds during actual athletic performances exceed 100 degrees per second.

Most of the isokinetic machines also have readout devices for recording muscle tension. This is a particular advantage since it provides for evaluation and may serve as a training monitor during actual training sessions.

A review of the types of muscular contractions is given in Figure 2–11.

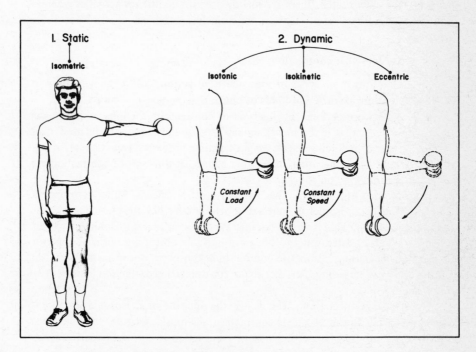

Figure 2–11. The four basic types of muscular contraction.

---

*For example, Cybex equipment from Lumex, Inc., Bayshore, NY 11706; and Mini-Gym equipment from Mini-Gym Inc., Independence, MO 65051.

3 □ Endurance Fitness Programs

As a reminder, cardiorespiratory or endurance fitness is defined as the capacity or ability of the heart-lung system to deliver blood and thus oxygen to the working muscles during prolonged physical exercise. In this chapter, we will address two major questions: (1) How does an endurance exercise program increase your fitness and simultaneously reduce your risk of coronary heart disease? and, (2) How often, how long, and how hard do you need to exercise in order to increase your endurance fitness level?

PHYSIOLOGICAL AND OTHER CHANGES RESULTING FROM ENDURANCE FITNESS PROGRAMS

Table 3–1 lists several important changes that occur following an endurance training program. The details of such a program will be presented later in this chapter. Most of the changes listed in the table are thought to be responsible for increasing your endurance fitness level and, at the same time, for decreasing your risk of coronary heart disease. A brief word about each change seems warranted.

Improvement in the Oxygen Transport System

This results mainly from an increased ability of the heart muscle to pump greater amounts of blood per minute to the working muscles. From the last chapter, you will recall that this is called the cardiac output (see Figure 2–5, p. 23).

TABLE 3-1   Physiological and Other Changes Resulting from
Endurance Exercise Programs

PHYSIOLOGICAL AND OTHER TRAINING CHANGES
• Improvement in the oxygen transport system
• Increased ability of skeletal muscles to use oxygen
• Increased circulatory efficiency
• Increased blood vessel size and capillarization of the heart muscle
• Reduced possibility of blood clot (thrombosis)
• Reduced occurrence of cardiac dysrhythmias
• Improved tolerance to stress

• Reduction in other coronary heart disease risk factors
  – Decreased obesity
  – Decreased blood pressure
  – Decreased blood cholesterol levels

Increased Ability of Skeletal Muscles to Use Oxygen

Supplying the skeletal muscles with more oxygen would not necessarily enhance their capacity for aerobic metabolism if their ability to use the oxygen were not also improved. This improvement in the use of oxygen is related mainly to biochemical changes that occur within the muscles cells.

Increased Circulatory Efficiency

The amount of blood pumped by the heart in one minute (the cardiac output) is affected by two major factors: (1) the amount of blood pumped by the heart with each stroke or beat (the stroke volume); and (2) the number of times the heart beats in one minute (the heart rate). Therefore, in order to pump a certain amount of blood each minute, the heart rate can be high and the stroke volume low or the heart rate can be low and the stroke volume high. In either case, the heart muscle, like any other muscle, requires energy, and thus oxygen, in order to perform its work. However, when the same amount of blood is pumped by the heart in one minute when the heart rate is low and the stroke volume high, less energy and thus less oxygen are required by the heart muscle itself than when the heart rate is high and the stroke volume low. In other words, the heart muscle can perform the same amount of work but with a lesser energy requirement when the heart rate is low and the stroke volume high. After training, circulatory efficiency increases because the same work is accomplished by the heart muscle but with a lowered energy requirement due to a decreased heart rate and increased stroke volume.

Increased Blood Vessel Size and Capillarization of the Heart Muscle

It is thought that the blood vessels of the heart increase in size following endurance training. This, of course, would enhance the blood flow and consequently the delivery of oxygen to the heart muscle. Aside from this change, there is also the possibility that endurance training leads to an increase in the number of vessels (particularly capillaries) that supply the heart muscle. This too would enhance blood flow and thus the delivery of oxygen to the heart.

Reduced Possibility of Blood Clot (Thrombosis)

In Chapter 1, it was mentioned that a heart attack or stroke occurs when the blood flow to the heart muscle or to the brain, respectively, is blocked, such as would be the case when a blood clot lodges in an artery. The possibility of the formation of blood clots is reduced by endurance training, thereby resulting in a reduced risk of serious cardiovascular accidents such as heart attack and stroke.

Reduced Occurrence of Cardiac Dysrhythmias

Disturbances in the rhythm (beating) of the heart (cardiac dysrhythmias) can lead to serious cardiac problems, including heart attack and death. It is thought that endurance training may reduce the susceptibility of the heart to such disturbances.

Improved Tolerance to Stress

Regular exercise training can lead to an improved tolerance to stress and a reduction in anxiety.

Reduction in Other Coronary Heart Disease Risk Factors

Regular exercise training leads to reductions in other coronary risk factors such as (a) decreased obesity; (b) decreased blood pressure; and (c) decreased blood cholesterol levels.

THE EXERCISE PRESCRIPTION

Now that we know how and why regular exercise training improves endurance fitness and reduces the risk of coronary heart disease, how should an endurance exercise program designed to do just that be constructed?

Medical Evaluation

Before starting your endurance exercise program, obtain your physician's approval. Although you may feel perfectly well and have never had any major medical problem, you still must see your physician and get his or her approval before beginning your program. It has been recommended that a medically supervised exercise "stress test" should be conducted on any adult 35 years of age or older before beginning an exercise program. Such a test is also mandatory for any person, regardless of age, who has a known cardiac condition (including one from which the person has recovered), occasional undiagnosed chest pain, or any of the major risk factors for coronary heart disease.

Quantity and Quality of the Exercise Program

The questions, "How much exercise is enough?" and "What type of exercise is best for developing and maintaining endurance fitness?" are frequently asked. There are four factors that must be considered in order to answer these questions: (1) the frequency of the endurance training program; (2) the intensity of the training program; (3) the duration of the training program; and (4) the mode of activity performed during the training program.

The American College of Sports Medicine makes the following recommendations for the quantity and quality of an exercise program for developing and maintaining endurance fitness in the healthy adult:

1. Frequency of Training. Exercise must be performed on a regular basis in order to assure improvement in your endurance fitness. Therefore, you should exercise three to five days per week, for example, on Monday, Wednesday, and Friday, or on Tuesday, Thursday, and Saturday, or Monday through Friday.

2. Intensity of Exercise. How do you know if you are exercising at the proper intensity? The best way is to know how high your heart rate is during the exercise session. Your *target heart rate,* that is, the heart rate which, during exercise, will assure you that you are exercising at the proper intensity, depends mainly on your maximum heart rate or your age and to a lesser extent your present fitness level. During your exercise session, your target heart rate should be between 60 and 90 percent of your *maximum heart rate reserve.* The heart rate reserve is the percent difference between your resting and maximum heart rate, added to your resting heart rate. Your resting heart rate is fairly easy to obtain. Your heart rate at rest can be determined by counting your pulse at any of several arteries, for instance, at the wrist, the neck, or the temple (see Figure 3–1). Your maximum heart rate, however, is not easy to obtain. Direct determination of your maximum heart rate requires a graded exercise stress test performed on either a treadmill or bicycle ergometer (see Chapter 7). Without such a test, your maximum heart rate can be estimated from your age as given in Table 3–2. Knowing your resting and maximum heart rates, an example of how

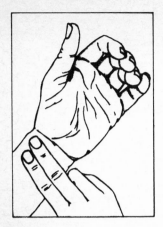
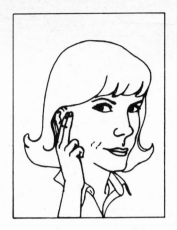
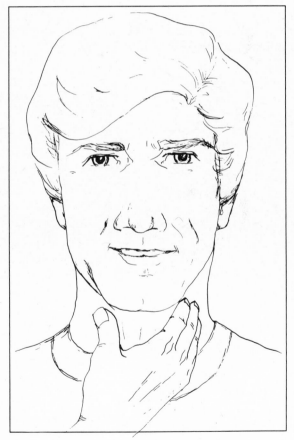

Figure 3-1. The heart rate may be determined by palpating the radial artery (at the wrist), the temporal artery (in front of the ear), or the carotid artery (in the neck).

TABLE 3–2 Estimated Maximum Heart Rates by Age*

AGE, YEARS	MAXIMUM HEART RATE, BEATS PER MINUTE
Less than 20	200
20 – 29	190
30 – 39	185
40 – 44	180
45 – 49	175
50 – 54	170
55 – 59	165
60 – 69	160
70 or greater	150 or less

*A "rule of thumb" for estimating your maximum heart rate is to subtract your age from 220. For example, if you are 35 years of age your maximum heart rate would be 220 – 35 = 185 beats per minute.

to calculate your exercise target heart rate (60 to 90 percent of your maximum heart rate reserve) is as follows:

Age   = 40 years
Resting heart rate   = 75 beats per minute
Estimated maximum heart rate (from Table 3–2) = 180 beats per minute
60% target heart rate   = $(180 - 75) \times 0.6 + 75$
                                                     = $105 \times 0.6 + 75$
                                                     = $63 + 75$
                                                     = *138 beats per minute*

90% target heart rate   = $(180 - 75) \times 0.9 + 75$
                                                     = $105 \times 0.9 + 75$
                                                     = $94.5 + 75$
                                                     = *169 beats per minute*

This means that if you are 40 years of age, the exercise you perform should be hard enough to raise your heart rate to at least 138 beats per minute but not greater than 169 beats per minute.

Target heart rate limits have been calculated for you by age and are given in Table 3–3. As an example of how to use the table, if you are 20 years of age and have a resting heart rate of between 60 to 75 beats per minute, your 60 percent target heart rate would be 141 beats per minute and your 90 percent rate, 177 beats per minute. During your exercise sessions, your heart rate should be between these limits. At the beginning of your exercise training program, shoot for the lower or 60 percent limit of your target heart rate. As you progress and become more fit, you can increase your target heart rate toward the upper or 90 percent limit. Never exceed this upper limit.

Although women tend to have slightly higher heart rates than do men, the maximum rates presented in Table 3–3 are applicable to both sexes since they are only estimates. Whenever possible, a directly determined maximum heart rate should be used in calculating your target heart rate.

TABLE 3-3 Target Heart Rates by Age

RESTING HEART RATE	AGE, YEARS	TARGET HEART RATE 60%	90%
	Less than 20		
75 – 90		153	188
60 – 75		147	186
45 – 60		141	185
	20 – 29		
75 – 90		147	179
60 – 75		141	177
45 – 60		135	176
	30 – 39		
75 – 90		144	175
60 – 75		138	173
45 – 60		132	171
	40 – 44		
75 – 90		141	170
60 – 75		135	168
45 – 60		129	166
	45 – 49		
75 – 90		138	166
60 – 75		132	164
45 – 60		126	162
	50 – 54		
75 – 90		135	161
60 – 75		129	159
45 – 60		123	158
	55 – 59		
75 – 90		132	157
60 – 75		126	155
45 – 60		120	153
	60 – 69		
75 – 90		129	152
60 – 75		123	150
45 – 60		117	149
	70 or older		
75 – 90		123	143
60 – 75		117	142
45 – 60		111	140

In order to check whether you are attaining your predetermined target heart rate, it is a good idea to occasionally take your pulse during the training sessions. Although it is not possible to take the pulse accurately during exercise, the pulse count obtained in a 6- or 10-second span immediately following exercise is a reasonable indicator of what the heart rate was during exercise. Remember, a 6-second count would be multiplied by 10, and a 10-second count by 6 in order to convert to beats per minute. For example, if you count 14 beats in 6 seconds, that would be 14 × 10 = 140 beats per minute. If you count 25 beats in 10 seconds, that would be 25 × 6 = 150 beats per minute. You will need to check your target heart rate at least once each week.

3. Duration of Exercise. During your workout, the exercise should be performed continuously at the proper intensity for 15 to 60 minutes per day. Duration is dependent on the intensity of the activity, thus lower intensity activities should be conducted over a longer period of time. A lower to moderate intensity activity of longer duration, as opposed to a higher intensity activity of shorter duration, is recommended for the nonathletic adult, that is, exercise at a target heart rate of 70 percent of the heart rate reserve for 60 minutes rather than at a training heart rate of 90 percent of the heart rate reserve for 15 minutes.

4. Mode of Exercise. The type of exercise to be used during your training program should have the following characteristics: (a) involves large muscle groups (e.g., the legs); (b) can be maintained continuously; and (c) is rhythmical and aerobic in nature. Examples of exercises fitting these characteristics are:

- running—jogging
- walking—hiking
- swimming
- skating (both ice and roller skating)
- bicycling (both on the open road and on an ergometer)
- rowing (actual or simulated)
- cross-country skiing
- rope skipping
- dancing (aerobic, ballet, and disco dancing)
- bench stepping

The selection of the proper activity is important in that it provides motivation for the participant to continue exercising on a regular basis.

Undoubtedly, the most popular modes of exercise are walking, jogging, and running, although bicycling and swimming are also very popular. At any rate, note from the above discussion that the duration, or how long you work out, is based on time, that is, 15 to 60 minutes, not on the completion of a certain number of miles. Because of this, the total distance covered during your workout depends upon how intensive the exercise needs to be in order to raise your heart rate to the target level. For example, if you need only to walk at 4 miles per hour in order to reach your target heart rate, then the distance covered in one workout will be between 1 and 4 miles.* If you need to jog at 6 miles per hour in order to obtain your target heart rate, then in 15 minutes you will have covered 1.5 miles and in 60 minutes, 6 miles.

You can tell at what speed you are walking or jogging by knowing how long it takes you to cover one mile. If you are just starting on a program, go to a track for the first week or so of your program. After you have established a pace that raises your heart rate to the target level, clock yourself to see how fast you are walking or jogging. After that, you can run over natural terrain and by knowing how long you have run, you will know approximately how far you have run.

---

*Fifteen minutes of walking at 4 miles per hour = 1 mile; 60 minutes of walking at 4 miles per hour = 4 miles.

TABLE 3-4   Distance Covered and Time per Mile while
Walking/Running at Various Speeds

MILES PER HOUR	MILES COVERED IN				MINUTES: Seconds per Mile
	15 min	30 min	45 min	60 min	
3.0	³/₄	1¹/₂	2¹/₄	3	20:00
3.5	⁷/₈	1³/₄	2²/₃	3.5	17:08
4.0	1.0	2.0	3.0	4.0	15:00
4.5	1¹/₈	2¹/₄	3³/₈	4.5	13:20
5.0	1¹/₄	2¹/₂	3³/₄	5.0	12:00
5.5	1³/₈	2³/₄	4¹/₈	5.5	10:54
6.0	1¹/₂	3.0	4¹/₂	6.0	10:00
6.5	1⁵/₈	3¹/₄	4⁷/₈	6.5	9:14
7.0	1³/₄	3¹/₂	5¹/₄	7.0	8:34
7.5	1⁷/₈	3³/₄	5⁵/₈	7.5	8:00
8.0	2.0	4.0	6.0	8.0	7:30
8.5	2¹/₈	4¹/₄	6³/₈	8.5	7:04
9.0	2¹/₄	4¹/₂	6³/₄	9.0	6:40
9.5	2³/₈	4³/₄	7¹/₈	9.5	6:19
10.0	2¹/₂	5.0	7¹/₂	10.0	6:00

A summary of the distance run or walked at various speeds and the corresponding time per mile is given in Table 3-4.

Various endurance game activities are also suitable as an exercise mode provided they fit the above characteristics. Tennis, for example, when played well, can be an effective endurance conditioner. Handball, racketball, paddle ball, and badminton can also be effective exercise modes provided they are played vigorously and on a regular basis.

A summary of the quantity and quality of the endurance exercise program for healthy adults is given in Table 3-5. It should be re-emphasized here that such a program is for *healthy* adults. Individuals who have symptoms of cardiovascular disease and/or for whom a complete exercise program is not medically advised should be placed in a modified program.

TABLE 3-5   Summary of the Quantity and Quality of Endurance
Exercise Programs for Healthy Adults*

Frequency of training	3 to 5 days per week
Intensity of training	Target heart rate of 60% to 90% of the heart rate reserve
Duration of training	15 to 60 minutes of continuous activity at the target heart rate
Mode of activity	Any activity that uses large muscle groups, that can be maintained continuously, and is rhythmical and aerobic in nature

*As recommended by the American College of Sports Medicine

Warm-up and Warm-down

Prior to starting a workout session, you should warm up, then following the workout, warm down. Three types of warm-up and/or warm-down activities are generally recommended: (1) stretching exercises for flexibility and for possible protection against muscular injury and soreness; (2) calisthenics for development of muscular strength and endurance; and (3) brief formal activity of the type used in your aerobic program. Of these three activities, the first one, stretching, should be considered the most important for the warm-up, whereas the first and third are best for the warm-down. Stretching exercises should be used that include most of the major muscle groups and joints of the body, that is, the neck, back, upper and lower legs, chest, hips, groin, spine, shoulders, arms, ankles, stomach, and feet. Each stretching exercise should be repeated five or six times and performed without bobbing or jerking and with the final stretched position held for 20 to 30 seconds. The following stretching exercises are only suggestions. Many other stretching exercises may be used with the same general results.

1. Achilles Tendon (Heel) and Gastrocnemius (Calf or Lower Leg). As shown in Figure 3–2, stand several feet in front of a wall with the feet several inches apart. Place outstretched hands on the wall, keeping the feet flat on the floor. Gradually move away from the wall by backing up but keep the feet flat on the floor. Hold the final stretched position. Each day try to increase the distance you move from the wall.

2. Neck. For stretching the neck, rotate the head, first in one direction, then in the other. Rotate slowly and repeat several times.

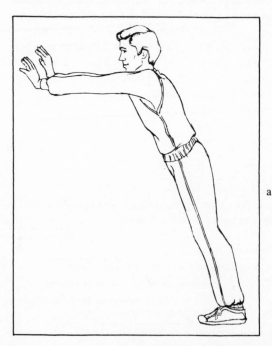

Figure 3–2. Achilles tendon and gastrocnemius stretch.

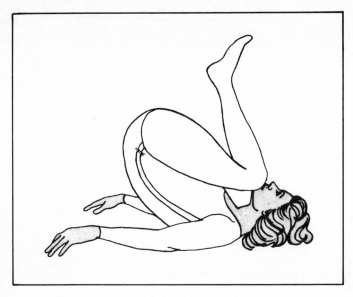

Figure 3-3. Back stretch.

3. Back (Figure 3-3). Lying on the back with the arms extended to the sides, bring the knees toward the chin as far as possible without raising the arms off the floor. Hold this position, then repeat.

4. Hamstrings (Back of Upper Leg). Sitting on the floor with legs spread, first reach for one foot, hold, then reach for the other foot and hold (Figure 3-4). Each time you reach, attempt to touch and hold the head and chest as close as possible to the thigh of the leg you are trying to hold at the foot. Repeat, reaching first for one foot and then the other.

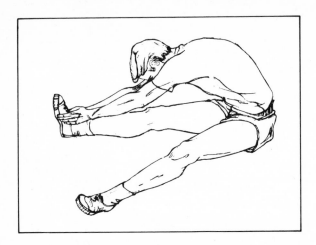

Figure 3-4. Hamstring stretch.

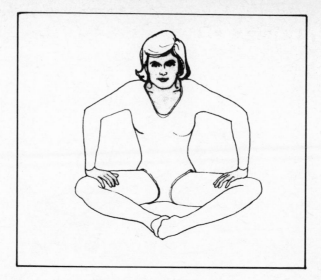

Figure 3–5. Groin stretch.

    5. Groin (Figure 3–5). Sit on the floor with the soles of the feet touching in front of you. Gradually push down on the knees as far as possible. Hold the final stretched position. Each day try to push the knees closer to the floor.

    6. Spine, Waistline (Figure 3–6). Sit on the floor with the right leg straight and cross it with the left leg, placing the left foot flat on the floor. With the right hand, reach around the left leg toward your left hip. Put the left arm directly behind you and slowly turn the head. Sit up straight, looking over the left shoulder. Hold, then stretch the other side by crossing the right leg over the left.

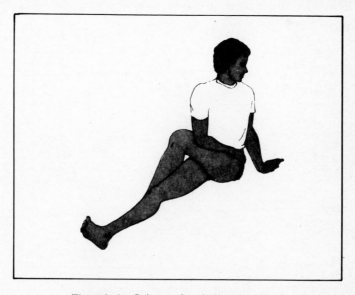

Figure 3–6. Spine and waistline stretch.

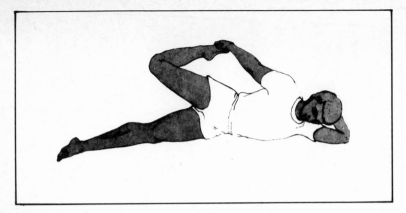

Figure 3–7. Quadriceps stretch.

7. Quadriceps (Front of Upper Leg). Lying on your left side, flex the knee of your right leg and grab the ankle with the right hand (Figure 3–7). Gradually move the hips forward until a good stretch is felt on the thigh. Hold. Repeat for the left leg by lying on your right side.

8. Shoulder, Chest (Figure 3–8). Stand with the feet several inches apart, with hands in front and the elbows raised to the side. Keep the head up and pull the elbows back as far as possible and hold. Repeat several times.

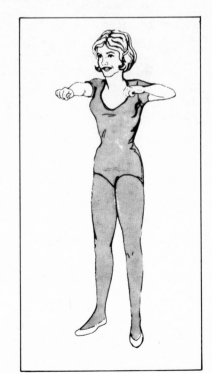

Figure 3–8. Shoulder and chest stretch.

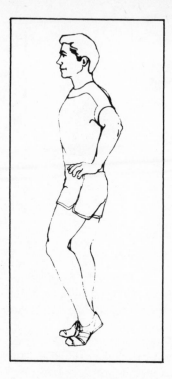

Figure 3–9. Ankle stretch.

9. **Ankle** (Figure 3–9). Standing with the weight on the right foot, place the ball of the left foot on the floor, transferring the weight to it gradually. Alternate by placing the ball of the right foot on the floor and transferring the weight to it from the left foot. Gradually increase the tempo to a jog.

10. **Abdominals** (Figure 3–10). Kneel by placing the hands and knees on the floor. Lean back onto the heels, extend the arms and place the chest on the floor. Hold, then repeat several times.

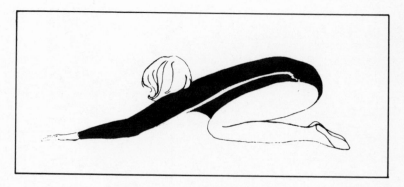

Figure 3–10. Abdominal stretch.

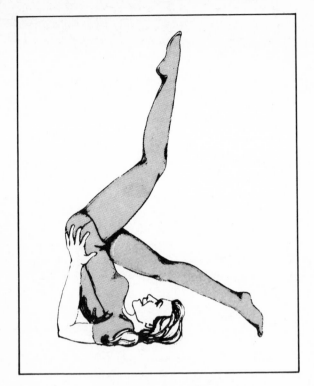

Figure 3–11. Hip stretch.

11. Hips (Figure 3–11). Lie on the back and raise the feet straight into the air, supporting the hips with the hands. Point the toes and touch first one foot to the floor above the head, hold, then do the same with the other foot. Repeat.

Improvement in muscular strength and muscular endurance of the legs usually will accompany your endurance exercise program since most of the activities involve the large leg muscles. Therefore, exercises for improving muscular strength and endurance should concentrate on the upper body, that is, the neck, abdomen, arms, and shoulders. Either calisthenics or weight resistance exercises may be used for this purpose (see Chapter 4).

The stretching exercises and formal activity used for the warm-down prevents the blood from pooling in the extremities, thus reducing the possibilities of dizziness and even fainting. Also, severe muscular soreness may sometimes be reduced as a result of the warm-down.

A Word About the Weather

Because endurance fitness programs involve activities that are performed continuously for up to one hour, a great deal of body heat is produced. Sweating is the body's main mechanism for losing heat. Two major problems can occur under these circumstances: (1) *dehydration* due to profuse sweating; and (2) *heat illness* due to overheating. If the activity is performed out of doors on a hot, humid day, these problems are greatly compounded. Dehydration and heat illness are characterized by such symptoms as weakness, exhaustion, headache, nausea, and if severe enough, cessation of sweating, collapse, confusion, and even death. Here are some guidelines on how to avoid such a tragedy:

1. Drink Plenty of Water. This is best accomplished by drinking small amounts (3 to 6 ounces) frequently. The drinking of large amounts of water at one time may make you feel uncomfortable. Salt tablets are *not* recommended. You should drink water before, during, and following your workout.

2. Wear Appropriate Clothing. Sweatsuits of any kind should *not* be worn under any circumstances when you are exercising in hot weather. This is an extremely dangerous practice that can cause death from overheating (*hyperthermia*). Contrary to popular belief, wearing sweatsuits in hot weather during exercise sessions does *not* promote the loss of body fat, but rather body water, which, as just emphasized, promotes dehydration and heat illness.

3. Work Out During the Coolest Part of the Day. The coolest parts of the day are in the morning and evening when the sun is "low" in the sky. On extremely hot and humid days, don't be afraid to cut back or skip your workout altogether.

Exercising in cold weather does not usually present a serious problem. This is so because adequate clothing for heat conservation and for protection against frostbite can (and should) be worn, and as was just mentioned, exercise increases body heat production.

Tips on Starting Your Endurance Program

The following tips may be helpful in getting a good start on your endurance training program:

- *First,* before starting your endurance fitness program, obtain your physician's approval.
- *Second,* start slowly. Don't be overly anxious in starting. Too often, the fast starters end up quitting first because of muscular soreness or chronic fatigue. Give your body a chance to adjust to the exercise. For most of you, only several days, or at most, a week will be all that is needed. Some muscular soreness is to be expected, but if it does not disappear after several weeks, consult your physician.
- *Third,* before exercising, don't forget to warm up with stretching exercises, particularly for those muscles you will be using during exercise.
- *Fourth,* stick with it. The benefits of exercise can be realized only if you exercise properly and on a regular basis. You can't expect improvement if you exercise one day the first week, two the second, none the third, and so on.

- *Fifth,* you should always end your exercise sessions with a warm-down or cool-down period of 5 or 10 minutes in which you gradually decrease your efforts before completely stopping. As mentioned earlier, a good warm-down activity is stretching.
- *Sixth,* exercise must be stopped if you experience one or more of the following warning signs:
  - Uncomfortable pressure, fullness, squeezing, or pain in the center of the chest or in the shoulder, neck, jaw, or arm.
  - Severe pain of any kind (e.g., leg cramps).
  - Dizziness.
  - Light-headedness (fainting).
  - Shortness of breath or rapid, distressful breathing.
  - Sudden weakness or numbness of the face, arm, or leg.
  - Sudden unsteadiness.
  - Sudden dimness or loss of vision.
  - Sudden loss of speech or trouble in speaking or understanding speech.
  - Unusual fatigue.
  - Lowering of your heart rate with increased exercise demands.
  - Fluttering in the chest (palpitations).

If any of these symptoms does not go away after exercise is stopped, get medical assistance immediately.

4 □ Muscular Fitness Programs

In Chapter 1, we defined muscular fitness as having three subcomponents: (a) *muscular strength*, which is defined as the force a muscle or muscle group can exert during contraction; (b) *muscular endurance*, defined as how long a period of time a muscle or muscle group can continue to exert force without fatiguing; and (c) *joint flexibility*, which is the range of motion possible at a joint over which a muscle spans. As in the previous chapter, the purpose of this chapter will be to answer two major questions concerning each of our muscular fitness components: (1) How do muscular fitness programs increase your strength, muscular endurance, and joint flexibility? and (2) How often, how long, and how hard do you need to exercise in order to increase your muscular fitness level?

PHYSIOLOGICAL AND OTHER CHANGES RESULTING FROM MUSCULAR FITNESS PROGRAMS

The most obvious effects of muscular fitness programs are increases in muscular strength, endurance, and flexibility. What causes these increases? What other changes occur as a result of muscular fitness programs? Let's see if we can answer some of these questions.

Table 4–1 lists some important physiological changes that are known to occur following muscular fitness programs or, more specifically, weight lifting programs. They are as follows:

Increased Muscle Size (Hypertrophy)

Of course, the most striking effect of weight lifting programs is an increase in the size of a muscle. In technical terms, this is called *hypertrophy*. It refers to an

46

TABLE 4-1   Summary of Physiological and Other Changes following
Muscular Fitness (Weight Lifting) Programs

PHYSIOLOGICAL OR OTHER CHANGES
Changes in Muscle Function Increased muscular strength Increased muscular endurance
Changes in Muscle Size Hypertrophy — increases in the diameters of existing fibers
Changes in Muscle and Joint Motion Increased flexibility or range of motion of a joint
Changes in Body Composition Decreased total and relative body fat Increased muscle mass (lean body weight)
Changes in Motor and Sports Skills Improved performance of some skills

increase in the diameter or cross-sectional area of the individual muscle fibers within a muscle. In other words, a muscle increases in size mainly as a result of increases in the size of existing fibers rather than by an increase in the number of fibers.*

Changes that contribute to increasing the size of the individual muscle fibers are: (1) increases in the number and the size of the myofibrils per muscle fiber; (2) increased amounts of the contractile proteins, actin and myosin; (3) increased numbers of capillaries supplying each fiber; and (4) increased amounts and strength of connective tissue, tendons, and ligaments. (To refresh your memory as to the structure of skeletal muscles, reread Chapter 2, pp. 24 to 27.) The increase in muscular endurance is probably related more to the third factor cited above rather than to some of the other factors.

It should be emphasized at this time that muscular hypertrophy is generally not as great in women as in men even when the same relative gain in strength has been made. Comparative measurements, such as those shown in Figure 4-1, bear this out. For example, as shown in the figure, the increases noted in girth or circumference of the muscles involved were, in every case, greater in men than in women. In addition, the largest increase in muscle size exhibited by the females (biceps or upper arm, chest and shoulders) was 0.6 centimeter, or less than a quarter of an inch! Such small increases in muscle size clearly demonstrate that muscular hypertrophy in women as a result of weight training programs will certainly not lead to excessive muscular bulk or produce a "masculinizing" effect.

---

*In some animals that have been "weight trained," small increases in the number of fibers have been observed; however, this has not been observed in humans.

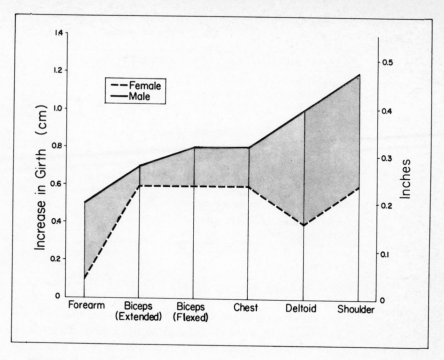

Figure 4–1. Increases in muscle size (hypertrophy) in females is generally not as great as that in males, even when the same relative gains in strength have been made.

Changes in Muscle and Joint Motion

An "old wives' tale" states that those who lift weights become "muscle bound" and thus immobile. Two points concerning this statement need clarification: First, weight lifting programs, when done properly, do not limit flexibility. In fact, such programs generally improve flexibility. Second, the term "muscle bound" is a misnomer in that hypertrophy of a muscle generally does not in itself limit the range of motion possible around the joint over which the muscle spans. In other words, there is no such concept as "muscle bound."

Changes in Body Composition

Generally, after weight training programs, total body weight either increases slightly or, in some instances stays the same. However, even with no change in total body weight, there is a change in *body composition*. Body composition refers to the proportion of the body that is fat and the proportion that is muscle, or more accurately, *nonfat* or *lean body weight*. We will study more about body composition in a later chapter (p. 79). Right now, we need to understand that after a weight training program, you may expect, in both sexes, to find little change in total body weight, a loss of body fat, and a gain in muscle mass or lean body weight (see Figure 4–2).

Changes in Motor and Sports Skills

Another "old wives' tale" states that weight lifting has a negative effect on the performance of many motor or sports skills. This is not true. Research has demonstrated that specific motor skills such as speed in swimming, throwing, and sprinting can be significantly improved through weight training programs.

It should be noticed that muscular fitness programs do *not* lead to significant increases in cardiorespiratory or endurance fitness. As emphasized in the last chapter, this is best accomplished through specific endurance fitness programs.

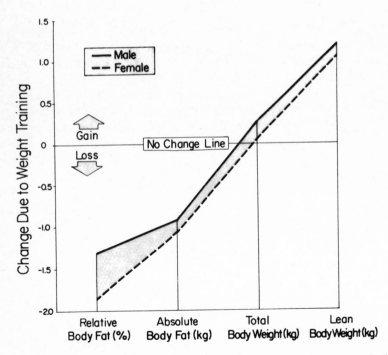

Figure 4–2. Following a weight training program you can expect, in both sexes, to find little change in total body weight, a loss of body fat, and a gain in muscle mass.

CONSTRUCTING MUSCULAR FITNESS PROGRAMS
(WEIGHT TRAINING PROGRAMS)

In Chapter 2, four basic types of muscular contractions were defined: isotonic, isometric, eccentric, and isokinetic. Weight resistance programs can be designed around each type of contraction. However, for our fitness purposes, only isotonic programs need to be considered. You will recall that an isotonic contraction is one in which the muscle shortens as it develops tension, such as when you lift a weight.

The best type of isotonic muscular fitness program involves what is referred to as either a *weight training, weight lifting,* or *weight resistance* program. Such programs consist of muscular contractions performed against resistance, as when lifting free weights (barbells) or weight stacks that are attached to specific weight lifting equipment such as Nautilus, Universal Gym, and other similar machines.

In order to properly construct your weight training program, several questions need answering: (1) How much weight should you lift? (2) How many days per week should you lift? and (3) Which muscle groups should you exercise and in what order?

How Much Weight Should You Lift?

One of the most important ingredients in your weight training program is the amount of weight lifted. This is as important to your weight training program as the target heart rate is to your endurance program. In order for a muscle to increase in strength and endurance, it must be *overloaded.* Overload, in this case, means to exercise the muscle against resistances that exceed those normally encountered. For example, a muscle that normally lifts 10 pounds on a regular basis needs to lift more than that in order to increase its strength and endurance. In other words, continuing to lift only 10 pounds will maintain the strength and endurance of the muscle but will not increase them. In the latter case, the muscle is said to be *underloaded* because it is being exercised against resistances normally encountered (see Figure 4–3).

Notice that the overload principle does not imply that the weights lifted must be extremely heavy, only that they be greater than those normally encountered. This is the key to a successful program, as lifting weights that are too heavy is a common mistake made by many people, particularly when they are just starting their program. Lifting extremely heavy weights, particularly at the beginning of your program is counter-productive and can lead to serious and sometimes permanent injury.

The proper weight to use when you first start is one with which you can do the exercise correctly for 15 repetitions. This weight will differ for each exercise, depending on the strength of the muscles. Each day, strive to increase the number of repetitions for the exercise, being careful to use correct form. When you are able to do 20 repetitions, increase the weight 5 pounds or one plate if you

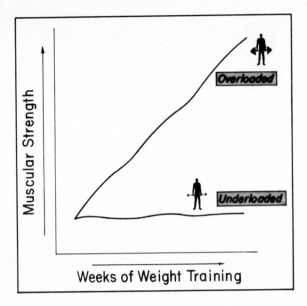

Figure 4–3. Muscular strength and endurance are most effectively developed when the muscle is overloaded — i.e., exercised against resistances exceeding those normally encountered. The strength and endurance of an underloaded muscle — one that is exercised against normally encountered resistance — will be maintained but not increased.

are using a machine with a weight stack. Do this for the first two weeks of training. It is perfectly normal for some muscle soreness and tightness to occur during the first few weeks of training, but this will soon disappear. The weights used will not be heavy enough to cause any injury. After two weeks, use a weight you can properly handle for 8 to 10 repetitions, and do not increase the weight until you can do 12 to 15 repetitions.

This latter point is another important part of your weight training program. It relates to the overload concept referred to earlier. Since an overloaded muscle gains in strength and endurance during the course of a weight training program, the initial overload (weight lifted) will, sometime later in the program, no longer provide adequate overload for continued gains in strength and endurance. In other words, the original overload eventually becomes an underload as strength and endurance are gained. For this reason, the resistance against which the muscle is exercised must be increased periodically throughout the course of the weight training program. One way to judge when a new overload should be introduced is to count the number of times a given weight can be lifted properly before fatigue sets in. From our above example, during the third week of your program, a weight should be selected that can be lifted properly 8 to 10 times. This amount of overload should then be used until you can perform 12 to 15 lifts. At that time, increase the load to such a degree that the number of repetitions to

the point of fatigue is once again reduced to 8 to 10. This pattern should be repeated as often as required throughout the duration of the program. In this
manner, the muscle will always work in the overload zone. Programs that in-
corporate this concept are called *progressive resistance programs.*

How do you select a weight that you can lift a certain number of times?
There is no easy way to do this. The simplest way is the good old trial and error
method. Start with light or moderate weight. If more than the required number
of repetitions can be performed, rest awhile, then add some weight (e.g., 10
pounds), and try again. Continue until the proper weight is selected. By the way,
this can be done with barbells or with any weight machine.

In summary, remember:

Your muscles must be overloaded, that is, they must be exercised against
resistances exceeding those normally encountered.

The overload must be progressive throughout the duration of the training
program.

During the first two weeks of your program, select a weight (by trial and
error) that you can correctly lift 15 times before your muscles fatigue. When
you reach 20 repetitions, increase the weight by 5 or 10 pounds.

After the second week, work with a weight you can lift 8 or 10 times before
fatiguing. When you reach 12 or 15 repetitions, increase the weight so that only
8 or 10 repetitions can again be performed.

How Many Days per Week Should You Lift?

Your weight training program should be conducted no more than three days
per week with a rest day between each workout. An example would be to work
out on Monday, Wednesday, and Friday and rest on Tuesday, Thursday, and the
weekend. Frequencies greater than this may cause chronic fatigue. If you are
also participating in an endurance fitness program, both programs may be performed on the same days but the weight training program should probably be
performed first.

Which Muscle Groups Should You Exercise?

Your weight training program should be well rounded and include exercises
for all the major muscle groups. These groups include: (1) upper legs and hips;
(2) chest and upper arms; (3) back and posterior (back) aspects of the legs;
(4) lower legs and ankles; (5) shoulders and posterior aspects of the upper arms;
(6) stomach (abdominals); and (7) anterior (front) aspects of the upper arms.
You should perform the exercises in the order given. In other words, as shown in
Figure 4-4, the exercises should be arranged so that the larger muscle groups are
exercised before the smaller ones. The reason for this arrangement is that smaller
muscles tend to fatigue sooner and more easily than do larger groups. Therefore,

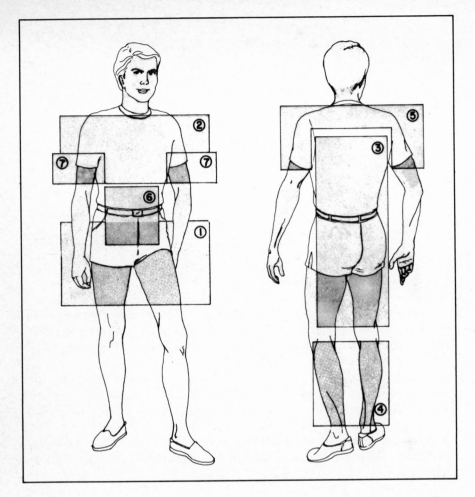

Figure 4–4. The order in which the major muscle groups should be exercised. The larger muscle groups should be exercised first. Code: **1**, upper legs and hips; **2**, chest and upper arms; **3**, back and posterior aspects of legs; **4**, lower legs and ankles; **5**, shoulders and posterior aspect of upper arms; **6**, abdomen; and **7**, anterior aspect of upper arms.

in order to ensure proper overload of the larger muscles, they should be exercised first, before the smaller ones fatigue.

Which Exercises Should You Do?

The specific exercises for the muscle groups outlined above and shown in Figure 4–4 are presented in Table 4–2. Notice that there is, for some muscle

TABLE 4-2 Weight-Training Exercises for Various Muscle Groups

MUSCLE GROUP	EXERCISE
Upper legs and hips	Leg curl, squats
Chest and upper arms	Bent-arm pullover, bench press, incline press, and arm curl
Back and posterior aspects of legs	Squats, stiff-legged dead lift, back hyperextension
Lower legs and ankles	Heel (toe) raises, squats
Shoulders and posterior aspects of upper arms	Bent-over row, press behind neck, pulldown (lat) machine, triceps extension
Abdomen (stomach)	Bent-knee sit-ups
Anterior aspects of upper arms and wrists*	Arm curls, wrist curls, wrist rollers

*Although the wrist muscles have not been previously mentioned, it is a good idea to include them in this group.

groups, more than one exercise that involves that particular group of muscles. In this case, only one exercise should be performed during any one workout. However, the exercises involving the same muscle groups may be substituted for each other on alternate days. An example of such a schedule is presented in Table 4-3.

Remember, for the first two weeks of your program, the weight for each exercise should be such that you can lift it at least 15 times but not more than 20. After the first two weeks, select a weight for each exercise that can be lifted 8 or 10 times. Work with that weight until 12 or 15 repetitions can be performed, then increase the weight until only 8 or 10 repetitions can again be performed. The one exception to this rule is with the bent-knee sit-ups. For this

TABLE 4-3 Weekly Schedule for Weight Training Exercises

MONDAY	WEDNESDAY	FRIDAY
Leg curl	Squat	Leg curl
Bent-arm pullover	Bench press/incline press*	Bent-arm pullover
Back hyperextension	Stiff-legged dead lift	Back hyperextension
Heel (toe) raises	Heel (toe) raises	Heel (toe) raises
Bent-over rowing/ Press behind neck*	Pulldown (lat) machine/ triceps extension*	Bent-over rowing/ Press behind neck*
Bent-knee sit-ups	Bent-knee sit-ups	Bent-knee sit-ups
Arm curls	Arm curls	Arm curls
Wrist roller	Wrist curl	Wrist roller

*Do one exercise or the other, but not both in the same workout.

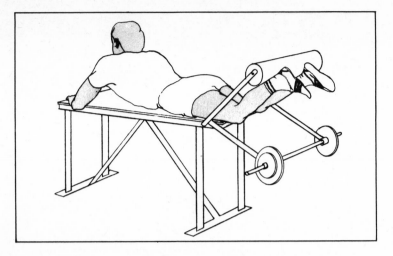

Figure 4-5. Leg curl.

exercise, work until you can perform 20 repetitions. Once 20 repetitions have been reached, hold a 2½- to 5-pound free weight on your chest to increase the resistance. Work with this weight until 20 repetitions can once again be performed, then increase the weight once again. You may want someone to hold your feet on the floor while you do your sit-ups.

Here are how the exercises are performed:

Exercises for the Upper Legs and Hips

Leg curl (Figure 4-5)

This exercise is performed with a leg machine. Lie face down on the edge of a table or leg machine. Flex your knees as far as possible and return. Repeat the required number of times.

Squat (Figure 4-6)

This exercise is performed with a barbell. Standing erect, place the barbell on your shoulders behind the neck. Your hands should be in a pronated (palms down) grip* and far apart. Keeping the back straight, lower the weight by flexing your knees to a 90° angle and return. Repeat the required number of times.

---

*A pronated grip refers to gripping the bar with the palms of the hands facing down.

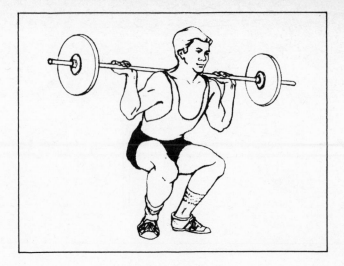

Figure 4–6. Squat.

Exercises for the Chest and Upper Arms

Bent-arm pullover (Figure 4–7)

This exercise is performed with a barbell. Lie on your back on a bench, holding the barbell over your head with elbows at a 90° angle and your hands in a

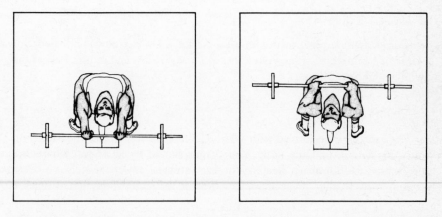

Figure 4–7. Bent-arm pullover. The grip shown here is called a pronated or palms-down grip.

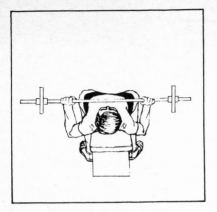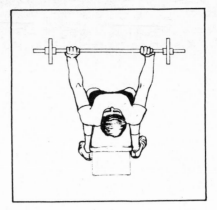

Figure 4–8. Bench press.

pronated (palms down) grip about shoulder-width apart. Lower the barbell over and behind your head as far as possible. Return to the starting position and repeat the required number of times.

Bench press (Figure 4–8)

This exercise is performed with a barbell. Lie on your back on a bench, holding the barbell over your chest with the arms extended, shoulder-width apart, and the hands in a pronated (palms down) grip. Lower the barbell to the chest and return. Repeat the required number of times.

Incline press

This exercise is a bench press (see above description) performed on an inclined bench (head raised above the feet).

Arm curl (Figure 4–9)

This exercise is performed with a barbell. From a standing position, hold the barbell in front of your thighs with your arms fully extended and your hands in a supinated* (palms up) grip. Raise the barbell to the chest by flexing the elbows. While lifting, stand erect and keep the elbows in toward the sides. Repeat the required number of times.

---

*A supinated grip refers to gripping the bar with the palms of the hands facing upward.

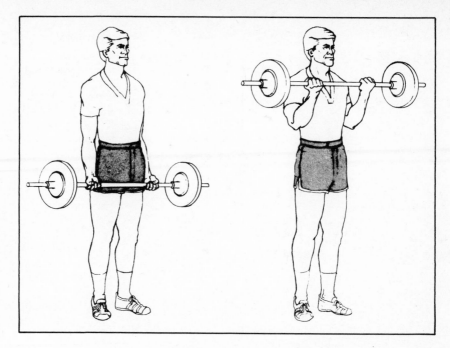

Figure 4–9. Arm curl.

Exercises for the Back and Posterior Aspects of the Legs

Squats

See p. 55.

Stiff-legged dead lift (Figure 4–10)

This exercise is performed with a barbell. Start from a standing position, holding the barbell in a pronated (palms down) grip with the arms extended and shoulder-width apart so that the barbell is resting in front of your thighs. With your knees locked, bend forward at the hips, lowering the barbell until it just touches the floor. Raise the weight by straightening the body. Repeat the required number of times.

Back hyperextension (Figure 4–11)

This exercise is performed with a free weight.* Lie face down with your upper body extending over the edge of a table and with a partner holding your legs.

---

*A free weight is just the weight, not the bar.

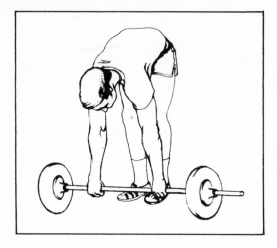

Figure 4–10. Stiff-legged dead lift.

Hold the weight behind your neck and lower your head toward the floor. On returning, raise your head and arch your back as much as possible. Repeat the required number of times.

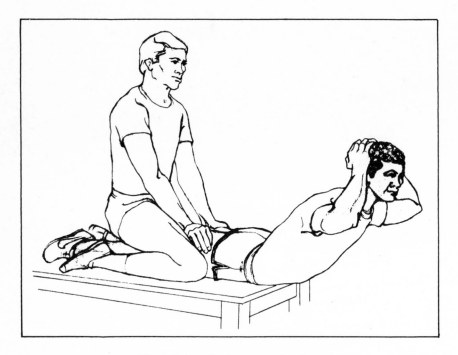

Figure 4–11. Back hyperextension.

Exercise for the Lower Legs and Ankles

Heel (toe) raise (Figure 4–12)

This exercise is performed with a barbell. With the barbell held across your shoulders and behind your neck, place the balls of your feet on a board about 2 inches high so that the heels are off the board. Rise up on the toes as far as possible, then lower the heels to the floor. Repeat the required number of times.

Exercises for the Shoulders and Posterior Aspects of the Upper Arms

Bent-over rowing (Figure 4–13)

This exercise is performed with a barbell. Flex your knees at a 45° angle and bend over from the hips until your back is parallel to the floor. With arms extended, grab the barbell with your hands pronated (palms down) and lift to the chest and return. Repeat the required number of times.

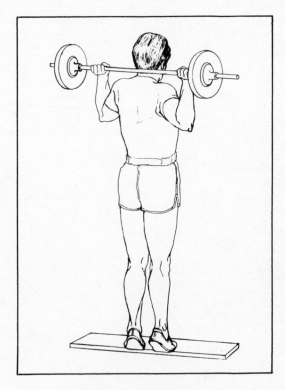

Figure 4–12. Heel (toe) raise.

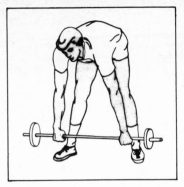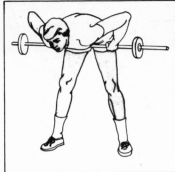

Figure 4–13. Bent-over rowing.

Press behind neck (Figure 4–14)

This exercise is performed with a barbell. Stand erect and hold the barbell behind your neck in a pronated (palms down) grip, with your hands about shoulder-width apart. Raise the weight overhead by fully extending your arms, then lower to behind the neck. Repeat the required number of times.

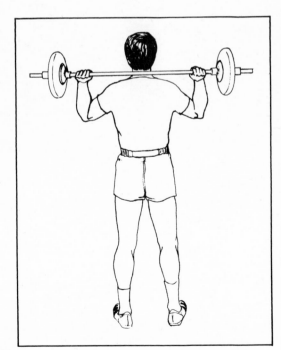

Figure 4–14. Press behind neck.

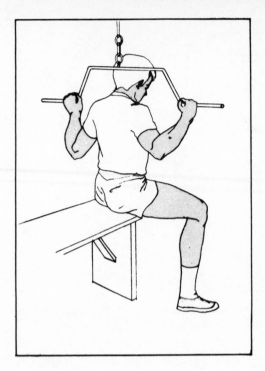

Figure 4–15. Pulldown lat machine.

Pulldown lat machine (Figure 4–15)

This exercise is performed with a lat machine. Sit on the end of a bench or kneel on the floor. Grasp the bar of the lat machine in a pronated (palms down) grip with your hands more than shoulder-width apart. Pull the bar down behind your head until it touches the base of the neck and shoulders. Return to the starting position and repeat the required number of times.

Triceps extension (Figure 4–16)

This exercise is performed with a lat machine. While standing, grasp the bar of the lat machine in a pronated (palms down) grip, keeping your hands closely together. The bar should be at about face level. Pull the bar downward as far as possible without bending your hips or knees. Return to the starting position and repeat the required number of times.

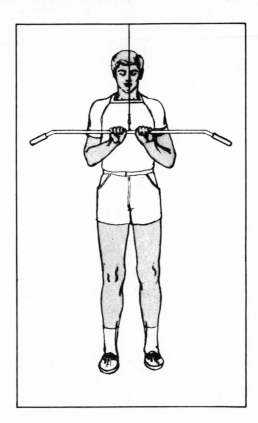

Figure 4-16. Triceps extension.

Exercise for the Abdomen (Stomach)

Bent-knee sit-ups (Figure 4–17)

Perform a regular sit-up but with the knees bent at approximately 90°.

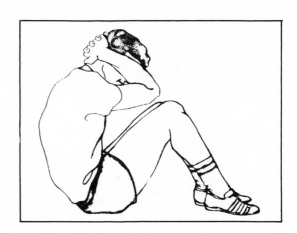

Figure 4-17. Bent-knee sit-up.

Exercises for the Anterior Aspects of the Upper Arms and Wrist

Arm curl

See p. 57.

Wrist curl (Figure 4–18)

This exercise is performed with a barbell. Grasp the barbell in a supinated (palms up) grip and sit with your forearms on your thighs so that your wrists and hands extend over your knees. Flex and extend your wrists as far as possible without raising your forearms from your thighs. Repeat the required number of times. To include the fingers, hold the barbell on the tips of your fingers with the hands open but cupped. Make a fist and then flex and extend the wrist.

Wrist roller (Figure 4–19)

This exercise is performed with a bar that has weights hanging on a rope from its center. While standing, grasp the bar in a pronated (palms down) grip and first raise the weights by rolling the rope up with the wrist and then lower the weights by unrolling the rope. Repeat the required number of times.

Barbells Versus Nautilus Versus Universal Gym

Probably the three most popular and familiar types of weight training equipment are barbells, Nautilus, and Universal. You may have noticed that most of the exercises just presented can be performed with barbells, although a few require special equipment such as that manufactured by Nautilus, Universal, and

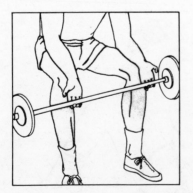
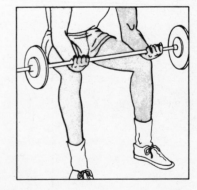

Figure 4–18. Wrist curl.

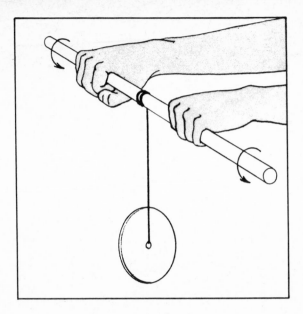

Figure 4–19. Wrist roller.

others. Without access to the various equipment, the program, as presented in Table 4–3, cannot be totally completed. Therefore, in Table 4–4, the exercises have been rearranged, again according to the muscle groups involved, but, in addition, also according to whether they can be performed with barbells, Nautilus machines, or the Universal Gym. For the Nautilus and Universal programs, both the name of the exercise and the name of the machine (in the case of Nautilus) and the name of the station (Universal) on which the exercises are performed are given. The three programs are equivalent to each other. Of course, if you have access to all of the necessary equipment and machines, you may wish to combine all three, choosing some exercises from each program. The same fundamental principles as discussed earlier apply equally to the three programs.

Flexibility through Weight Training

Earlier it was mentioned that the term "muscle bound" was a misnomer in that muscular bulk does not normally limit flexibility. Not only is it a misnomer but just the opposite effect is possible. In other words, an increase in flexibility is a common result of weight training programs that are done properly. Each exercise should be performed through the *full* range of motion. This will assure an increase in flexibility. Also, stretching exercises are similarly important in improving flexibility.

Table 4–4 Weight Training Exercises for Different Muscle Groups Using Barbells, Nautilus, or Universal Gym Equipment

MUSCLE GROUP	BARBELLS	UNIVERSAL Exercise	UNIVERSAL Equipment	NAUTILUS Exercise	NAUTILUS Equipment
Upper legs and hips	Squat	Leg press Leg curl Leg (knee) extension	Leg press station Thigh and knee machine	Super hip and back Duo-poly hip and back Leg extension Leg press Leg curl	Super geared hip and back machine Duo-poly hip and back machine Leg extension machine Compound leg machine Leg curl machine
Chest and upper arms	Bent-arm pullover Bench press Incline press	Pulldown or lat machine Bench press Dips	High lat pull station Chest press station Dipping station	Decline press bent-arm fly Pullover Duo-poly pullover Lat pulldown	Double chest machine Pullover machine Duo-poly pullover machine Torso arm
Back and posterior aspects of legs	Back hyperextension Stiff-legged dead lift	Back hyperextension Leg curl Stiff-legged dead lift	Back hyperextension Thigh and knee machine Quad and dead lift station	Super hip and back Duo-poly hip and back Leg curl	Super geared hip and back machine Duo-poly hip and back machine Leg curl machine
Lower legs and ankles	Heel (toe) raises	Heel (toe) raise	Leg press station	Heel (toe) raise	Multi-exercise machine

Body region					
Shoulders and posterior aspects of upper arms	Bent-over rowing Press behind neck	Chin-up Pulldown on lat machine Seated press Upright rowing Triceps extension	Chinning station High lat pull station Shoulder press station Quad and dead lift station High lat pull station	Pullover Lat pulldown Side lateral raise, seated press	Pullover machine Torso arm machine Double shoulder machine
Abdomen (stomach)	Bent-knee sit-up	Bent-knee sit-up Leg raise	Abdominal conditioner station Hip flexor station	Sit-up leg raise	Multi-exercise machine
Anterior aspects of upper arm	Arm curl	Arm curl Chin-up	Quad and dead lift station Chinning station	Chin-up Arm curl	Multi-exercise machine Omni bicep machine
Wrist (forearm)	Wrist curl Wrist roller	Wrist curl Wrist roller	Wrist and forearm station	Wrist curl	Multi-exercise machine

Warm up

A good time to do your stretching exercises for improving flexibility is right before you lift. In this way, the stretching exercises will serve two purposes: improve flexibility and provide a warm up for your lifting program. Some examples of stretching exercises were given in the last chapter.

Tips on Starting Your Weight Training Program

The following tips may be helpful in getting a good start on your muscular fitness program:

- *First,* avoid lifting extremely heavy weight. This will only cause injury and will eventually be counter-productive.
- *Second,* stick with the progressive overload plan as recommended here. Once again, during the first two weeks, select a weight that can be lifted 15 times. When 20 repetitions can be completed, add 5 pounds. After two weeks, use a weight that can be lifted 8 or 10 times. Work with this weight until you can perform 12 or 15 repetitions, then increase the weight so that only 8 or 10 repetitions can again be performed. If you are using barbells or Universal, try increasing the weight by 5 or 10 pounds. If you are using Nautilus, try to increase the weight by one plate. If, upon increasing the weight, you are unable to lift the minimum number of repetitions (8 or 10), return to the previous weight for two more workouts.
- *Third,* when performing any exercise, avoid what is referred to as "throwing" the weight by lifting or jerking the weight. Proper lifting involves moving the weight with a relatively slow steady movement. For example, when lifting a weight, count to three; when lowering a weight, count to four.
- *Fourth,* use correct form at all times. This means being able to lift without jerking or "struggling" with the weight and completing the lift through the full range of motion.
- *Fifth,* during the first two or three weeks, you should rest two minutes between each exercise. As you gain in strength, the two-minute rest period should decrease to one minute. Your total workout should take only 30 to 35 minutes to complete.

5 □ Nutritional Fitness Programs

Nutritional fitness, as defined in Chapter 1, is concerned with proper selection of foods with regard to their nutrient and caloric values as well as with proper eating habits. A nutritional fitness program is one in which all of these factors are practiced on a regular day-to-day basis. In this chapter, you will learn what food nutrients are, what your food requirements are, and what constitutes good or proper eating habits.

FOOD NUTRIENTS

There are three fundamental classes of food nutrients: (1) energy nutrients; (2) vitamins and minerals; and (3) water.

Energy Nutrients

Energy nutrients are those foods that, when chemically broken down, release energy, some of which is captured as ATP. You should recall from Chapter 2 that *proteins, fats,* and *carbohydrates* are the energy nutrient foods. Of these, the main energy nutrients are fats and carbohydrates (glucose and glycogen). The magnitude of the stores of these nutrients within the body is dependent to a great extent upon our diets.

Protein is not normally used as an energy nutrient, although it can and does serve as such under certain unusual circumstances (e.g., during starvation). The main contribution of protein is for cellular and tissue growth and repair in the body. Proteins are complex molecules containing *amino acids.* Some, but not all, of the essential amino acids are made by the body. Those that are not made by the body can only be obtained through the diet. Thus, the importance of daily dietary protein is obvious.

Some natural foods that are rich sources of the energy nutrients — fats, carbohydrates, and proteins — are listed in Table 5–1.

TABLE 5–1   Natural Foods in Each of the
Energy Nutrient Categories

FAT	CARBOHYDRATE	PROTEIN
Bacon	Baked beans	Cereal
Butter	Bread	Cheese
Margarine	Cakes	Eggs
Nuts	Cereals	Fish
Peanut butter	Dried fruits	Lean meat
Pork	Fresh fruits	Liver
Salad oils	Honey	Milk
	Pastries	Nuts
	Potatoes	Poultry
	Syrup	Soya beans
	Vegetables	Yeast (brewer's)
		Vegetables (legumes)

Vitamins and Minerals

Most vitamins serve as essential parts of enzymes or coenzymes that are vital to the metabolism of the energy nutrients. Thus, although vitamins do not in themselves yield energy, they are essential to life (i.e., they are nutrients).

Vitamins are classified as water soluble or fat soluble. The water-soluble vitamins are vitamin C (ascorbic acid) and the B-complex vitamins. These are *not* stored in the body and therefore must be constantly supplied in the diet. Since they are not stored, when taken in excess (more than the required amount), they will be passed in the urine. The fat-soluble vitamins, A, D, E, and K, *are* stored in the body, principally in the liver but also in fatty tissue. While this means that these vitamins need not be supplied each day, it also means that excessive accumulations can cause toxic effects.

A deficiency of vitamins can lead to serious illness, chronic disease, and even death. However, deficiencies, particularly in the United States, are very rare. The minimum daily requirements of vitamins are small and can be easily met through a varied diet. Although most fats, carbohydrates, and protein foods contain vitamins, the richest sources are green leafy vegetables (see Table 5–2).

Minerals are compounds that are found in trace amounts in the body and are also important to proper bodily function. Calcium, phosphorus, potassium, sodium, iron, and iodine are a few of the more important required minerals. Mineral deficiencies are generally uncommon today.

Although iodine is artificially added to common table salt ("iodized" salt is the result), most minerals occur naturally in a large variety of foods. For example, milk is rich in calcium, as are other dairy products, and in potassium, as are dried fruits and wheat germ. Most animal protein foods are good sources of phosphorus, and lean meats, particularly liver, provide enough iron to meet most dietary requirements. Common table salt supplies us with sodium.

TABLE 5-2 Fat-Soluble and Water-Soluble Vitamins
and Their Rich Food Sources*

VITAMIN	RICH FOOD SOURCE
Fat-Soluble Vitamins	
Vitamin A	Liver, egg yolk, milk, butter, yellow vegetables, greens
Vitamin D	Sunlight, fish, eggs, fortified dairy products
Vitamin E	Vegetable oils, greens
Vitamin K	Greens, liver
Water-Soluble Vitamins	
B-Complex Vitamins	
Vitamin B_1	Meat, whole grain cereals, milk, legumes (e.g., beans)
Vitamin B_2	Milk, fish, eggs, meat, green vegetables
Niacin	Peanut butter, whole-grain cereals, greens, meat, poultry, fish
Vitamin B_6	Whole-grain cereals, bananas, meats, spinach, cabbage, lima beans
Folic acid	Greens, mushrooms, liver
Vitamin B_{12}	Animal foods
Vitamin C	Citrus fruits, tomatoes, strawberries, potatoes, papaya, broccoli, cabbage

*Modified from Smith, N. J.: *Food for Sport.* Palo Alto, California: Bull Publishing Company, 1976.

Water

Of all the nutrients, water is probably the most essential for human life. For example, water makes up about 50 to 55 percent of our total body weight, 72 percent of our muscle weight, and 80 percent of our blood is water. While we can go without food for several months, we can survive only a matter of days without water. Water is important in the regulation of body temperature and it is the medium in which all the body processes occur (e.g., metabolic chemical reactions, exchange of oxygen and carbon dioxide, and so on).

The greatest sources of water intake are from drinking water and the water contained in beverages and soups. However, several food sources also contribute large quantities of water. For example, watermelon, broccoli, carrots, oranges, pineapple, potatoes, green beans, pickles, celery, and lettuce are more than 80 percent water.

As mentioned in Chapter 3 (p. 44), dehydration or the loss of body water is a serious problem that can lead to death. This is particularly true during exercise in hot, humid environments when large amounts of body water in the form of sweat are lost. The drinking of water under these conditions is mandatory.

FOOD REQUIREMENTS

Food requirements are dependent upon two factors: (1) nutritional needs and (2) caloric needs.

Nutritional Needs

No single nutrient should supply 100 percent of the caloric intake. Of the total *calories* taken in, a certain proportion should be derived from each of the three food nutrients discussed earlier:

- Protein: 10 to 15 percent
- Fat: 25 to 30 percent
- Carbohydrates: 55 to 60 percent

As an example, if your daily caloric requirement is 2500 kilocalories (kcal),* you should obtain 250 to 375 kcal from proteins, 625 to 750 kcal from fats, and 1375 to 1500 kcal from carbohydrates. In terms of weight rather than calories, this would be 2.0 to 3.0 ounces of protein, 2.5 to 3.0 ounces of fat, and 12 to 13 ounces of carbohydrates.

A word is needed here about the kind of fat that should be eaten. There are *saturated fats* and *unsaturated fats*. Consumption of large amounts of saturated fats is not recommended since this is thought to lead to high blood cholesterol levels, atherosclerosis, cardiovascular disease, and obesity. All of these factors, you will recall, are known coronary heart disease risk factors. Your fat intake then should consist primarily of unsaturated fats.

Saturated fats are usually in a solid form at room temperature. They include most of the animal fats, that is, the fats in meats such as beef, pork, or lamb. Eggs and dairy products also contain high levels of saturated fats. Unsaturated fats are in a liquid form at room temperature. They are found in vegetable oils such as peanut oil, corn oil, and soybean oil.

For most individuals, whether athletic or not, apportioning the diet along the lines given here should, under most circumstances, supply adequate amounts of the energy nutrients plus needed vitamins and minerals.

Caloric Needs

The calories that you take in as food should be approximately equal to the calories that you expend for body maintenance and physical activities. Thus, if

---

*A kilocalorie is a unit of work or energy equal to the amount of heat required to raise one kilogram (2.2 pounds) of water one degree centigrade (1.8 degrees Fahrenheit). It is abbreviated kcal.

you expend 2500 kcal daily, then you should take in 2500 kcal per day in order for your body weight to remain constant. An athlete may expend 5000 or even 7000 kcal per day during heavy training and competition. Replacing these calories requires a caloric intake of the same magnitude if the body weight is to be maintained. Caloric imbalance such as is required for gaining or losing weight will be discussed in the next chapter.

EATING HABITS

Good eating habits entail knowing how to select foods and how many meals to eat per day. It is most common to select specific foods from the following four food groups:

- Milk and milk products
- Meat and high-protein foods
- Fruits and vegetables
- Cereal and grain foods

Selection of foods from these four basic food groups will ensure a well-balanced diet from a nutritional standpoint. Table 5–3 gives examples of specific foods in these food groups, their minimum daily amounts, and their main nutritional contributions. Table 5–4 provides examples of a basic five-meal diet and a three-meal diet. Notice that the diets contain only 1200 to 1400 kcal — not nearly enough for most of us. However, the old saying, "First eat what you need and then eat what you want," is applicable here. What you need nutritionally is contained in these basic diets.

Ordinarily, three meals a day are eaten. These meals usually satisfy the normal caloric requirements of the nonathlete. However, the caloric requirements of athletes are frequently doubled during periods of heavy physical activity and it is recommended that under these circumstances, five to six meals a day be eaten. An example of an eating schedule for someone with a 2500 kcal requirement might look like this:

	kcal %	Total kcal
Breakfast	20.0	500
Lunch	35.0	875
Dinner	45.0	1125
Total	100.0	2500

A word about snacks is appropriate here. Snacking is perhaps one of the primary causes of obesity. However, "nutritive" snacking, that is, snacking on foods of nutritional value, can aid in the maintenance of proper blood glucose (sugar) levels and, at the same time, effectively fulfill the high caloric requirements of active people. "Junk foods," as foods without nutritional value are called, should be completely eliminated from the diet. Some examples of nutritive snacks are bananas, yogurt, fruit juices, sandwiches (e.g., peanut butter, bologna), dried fruit, malted milk, nuts, raisins, and oatmeal cookies.

TABLE 5-3   Daily Food Guide for the Four Basic Food Groups*

FOOD GROUP	DAILY AMOUNTS	MAIN CONTRIBUTION
I. Milk and cheese or equivalents†	Children under 9: 2 to 3 cups Children 9 to 12: 3 or more cups Teenagers: 4 or more cups Adults: 2 or more cups Pregnancy: 3 or more cups Lactation: 4 or more cups	Calcium Protein Riboflavin Vitamin D
II. Meat: Beef, veal, pork, lamb, poultry, fish, eggs Alternates: Dry beans, dry peas, lentils, nuts, peanut butter	2 or more servings Serving size: 2–3 ounces lean, boneless cooked meat, poultry, fish 2 eggs 1 cup cooked dry beans, dry peas or lentils 4 tablespoons peanut butter	Protein Thiamin Iron Niacin Riboflavin
III. Bread and cereals (whole-grain or enriched)	4 or more servings Serving size: 1 slice bread ½ to ¾ cup cooked cereal, macaroni, spaghetti, hominy grits, kasha, rice, noodles, bulgur 1 ounce (1 cup) ready-to-eat cereal 5 saltines or 2 graham crackers	Thiamin Riboflavin Niacin Iron Protein
IV. Vegetables and fruits	4 or more servings Serving size: ½ cup dark green or deep yellow every other day ½ cup or 1 medium citrus fruit (or any raw fruit or vegetable rich in ascorbic acid) Other vegetables and fruit including potato (1 medium)	 Vitamin A Ascorbic Acid Other vitamins and minerals
Water	6 to 8 glasses	

*From Krause, M., and Hunscher, M.: *Food, Nutrition and Diet Therapy*. 5th ed. Philadelphia: W. B. Saunders Company, 1972.

†Milk equivalents: 1 cup whole or skimmed milk, 1 cup buttermilk, ½ cup evaporated milk, ¼ cup nonfat milk powder, 1 ounce cheddar cheese, 2 cups ice cream, 1½ cups cottage cheese. (The amount given is figured on the basis of calcium content.)

Misunderstood Concepts Concerning Nutrition during Exercise and Training

Three misunderstood concepts concerning nutrition during exercise training and competition are the protein requirement, the use of supplemental vitamins and minerals, and what to eat before you exercise.

TABLE 5–4   Examples of Basic Diets in Three and Five Meals*

5 MEALS	3 MEALS
Breakfast ¹/₂ grapefruit ²/₃ cup bran flakes 1 cup skim or low-fat milk or other beverage	**Breakfast** ¹/₂ cup orange juice 1 soft-boiled or poached egg 1 slice whole wheat toast 1¹/₂ teasp. margarine 1 cup skim or low-fat milk or other beverage
Snack 1 small package raisins ¹/₂ bologna sandwich	
	Lunch 1¹/₂ cup Manhattan clam chowder 2 rye wafers ¹/₂ cup cottage cheese (uncreamed) 1 medium bunch grapes or 1 medium apple 1 granola cookie
Lunch 1 slice pizza 1 serving of carrot sticks 1 apple 1 cup skim or low-fat milk	
Snack 2 oatmeal cookies	
	Dinner 1 helping of oven-barbecued chicken (3 oz, no bone) ¹/₂ cup green beans ¹/₂ cup cabbage and carrot salad ²/₃ cup mashed potato ¹/₂ cup applesauce 1 cup skim or low-fat milk or other beverage
Dinner 1 baked fish with mushroom (3 oz) 1 baked potato 2 teasp. margarine ¹/₂ cup broccoli 1 cup tomato juice or skim or low-fat milk	
Total calories: about 1400	
	Total calories: about 1200

*From Smith, N. J.: *Food for Sport.* Palo Alto, California: Bull Publishing Co., 1976.

The protein requirement

The normal adult daily protein requirement is about 1 gram per kilogram of body weight. For example, the daily protein requirement of a person weighing 75 kg (165 pounds) would be 75 kg $\times$ 1 g/kg = 75 grams (2.6 ounces). This amount of protein is easily obtained from a well-balanced diet in which 10 to 15 percent of the calories taken in are from protein sources. If our 165-pound person has a daily caloric requirement of 3000 kcal, a well-balanced diet would supply between 75 and 112 grams of protein.* Contrary to what many coaches and athletes believe, the protein requirement during heavy exercise and training is not significantly increased in adults. Thus, the amount of protein sufficient to meet the body's ordinary demands will also be sufficient during periods of increased physical activity — even during heavy weight training involving increases in muscle mass.

---

*Ten percent of 3000 kcal = 300 kcal, and 15% = 450 kcal. One gram of protein contains 4 kcal. Therefore, 300/4 = 75 grams, and 450/4 = 112 grams of protein.

It should be noted that since the protein requirement is estimated on a body-weight basis, it provides for greater protein intake with increases in muscle mass. For example, an active male football player who weighs 115 kg (253 pounds) would have a daily protein requirement of 115 grams. If his daily caloric requirement were 5000 kcal, a well-balanced diet providing 10 to 15 percent of its calories in the form of protein would provide him with between 138 and 187 grams of protein. He would easily meet his requirement.

The consumption of excessive quantities of protein, particularly in the form of pills and powders, during heavy exercise and training is neither required nor recommended. In fact, it may be contraindicated in many sports since a diet excessively high in protein may cause dehydration.

Use of vitamin and mineral supplements

With respect to exercise, there does not appear to be an excessive demand for most vitamins or minerals during periods of increased physical activity. The one exception might be the requirement for iron, which is found in red blood cells and is responsible for the oxygen-carrying ability of the blood. Levels of iron in the blood of women have been found to be significantly decreased after heavy physical training; thus, women athletes, especially those who have heavy menstrual blood losses, may wish to consider supplementing their diets with extra iron. A note of caution is needed here: overdoses of iron can be toxic. Therefore, anyone contemplating taking iron supplements should first consult a physician.

Use of vitamin and mineral supplements is fairly common among athletes (as well as the general population). For example, it has been reported that 85 percent of the Olympic athletes use vitamin and mineral supplements. Although some of these athletes have indicated that the supplements have improved their performances, little scientific evidence is available to support their contentions. Furthermore, those authorities who recommend vitamin supplements for athletes usually do so only on theoretical grounds (the value of extra vitamins is inferred from the fact that meeting the basic vitamin requirement is essential to life).

It may be concluded that supplementing the diet with amounts of vitamins and minerals above the minimum daily requirements does not increase physical performance. Furthermore, the minimum daily requirements are easily met through a varied, normal diet.

What to eat before exercising or competing

From what has already been stated, you should realize that there are no foods that, when taken several hours prior to physical activity, will lead to "super" performances. Proper nutrition, as emphasized throughout, is a year-round task.

However, there are certain foods that should probably be avoided on the day of intense exercise or competition. For example, fats and meats are generally digested slowly. If consumed within four hours (or less) of an athletic event they may cause a feeling of fullness, thus hindering performance. Other food categories to avoid might include gas-forming foods, "greasy" foods, and highly seasoned foods.

Carbohydrates should be the major constituent of the so-called "pregame meal" and should be consumed no later than 2½ hours before exercising or competing. Carbohydrates are easily digested and help maintain the blood glucose (sugar) levels (the latter effect makes one "feel" better). The pregame meal can also include moderate portions of such foods as fruits, cooked vegetables, gelatin desserts, and fish (or lean meats, provided the advice given above is heeded).

Consumption of large amounts of sugar, particularly in liquid or pill form, less than an hour before exercise is not recommended. Such consumption, rather than making more sugar available to the muscle cells, actually reduces blood-borne sugar (glucose) during exercise. In turn, this places greater dependence upon the sugar (glycogen) stored in the muscle, and early fatigue can result.

Provided their sugar concentration is not excessive, liquids may (and should) be imbibed up to 30 minutes before physical activity, particularly long-term exercise. Water is perhaps the best liquid, but fruit and vegetable juices are suitable, as are uncarbonated fruit-flavored drinks.

What about coffee? Some of you may have heard that caffeine can increase your endurance performance. While this is true from a scientific viewpoint, you should not drink a lot of coffee in hopes of increasing your endurance performance. The side effects of caffeine and other ingredients of coffee are not yet known.

An increasingly popular pregame meal with both coaches and athletes is the liquid meal. There are several liquid formulae commercially available today that can serve as excellent pregame meals (e.g., Ensure, Ensure Plus, Nutriment, Sustagen, and SustaCal). Available in a variety of flavors to suit most tastes, liquid meals are well-balanced nutritionally (most contain large amounts of carbohydrates plus some fats and proteins). Besides being palatable and nutritious, liquid meals are easily digested and are emptied quickly from the stomach. As both a "liquid" and a "meal," they contribute to hydration and to energy intake. There are subjective effects as well: drinking a liquid meal will give you a feeling of satisfaction and relief from hunger. At the very least, the occasional unpleasant sensations associated with exercise or competition (nervous indigestion, diarrhea, nausea, vomiting, and abdominal cramps) are minimized when liquid meals are used.

It should be emphasized that what you eat before you exercise or compete is not entirely based on strict "do's" or "don'ts." The basic requirement is a relative one: your diet on the day of exercise or competition should not be drastically different from that which you normally consume (so long as it is remembered that nervousness and tension during intense competition may so affect the digestive system that the foods normally eaten without discomfort may now cause distress). Provided you do not overeat or do not eat foods that will cause gastrointestinal discomfort, performance will not be affected per se by the foods consumed on the day you exercise.

Guidelines to follow in planning what to eat before you exercise are given in Table 5–5.

TABLE 5–5   Guidelines to Follow in Planning What to Eat Before Exercising*

Energetics of the Diet
Energy intake should be adequate to ward off any feelings of hunger or weakness during the entire period of exercise. Although pre-contest food intakes make only a minor contribution to the immediate energy expenditure, they are essential for the support of an adequate level of blood sugar, or for avoiding the sensations of hunger and weakness.

Timing of the Diet
The diet plan should ensure that the stomach and upper bowel are empty at the time of exercise.

Fluid Content of the Diet
Food and fluid intakes prior to and during prolonged exercise should guarantee an optimal state of hydration.

Blandness of the Diet
The pre-exercise diet should offer foods that will minimize upset in the gastrointestinal tract.

Psychological Aspects of the Diet
The diet should include food that you are familiar with, and that you are convinced will "make you win."

*Recommendations under each heading are from Smith, N. J.: *Food for Sport.* Palo Alto, California: Bull Publishing Co., 1976.

6 □ Diet, Exercise, and Body Weight Control

In the previous chapter, the importance of good nutritional fitness was discussed, and in Chapters 3 and 4, the importance of good endurance and muscular fitness programs was discussed. In this chapter, the importance of both nutrition and regular exercise will be discussed as they affect body weight control. As mentioned in the first chapter, obesity or overfatness is a major health problem in the United States today. How serious is it? Over 50 percent of the adult population is overfat!

To understand how you can control your body weight, you need to know what body composition is and how it can safely and effectively be changed through diet and exercise.

BODY COMPOSITION

Body composition refers to the component parts of the body. For our purposes, the body may be regarded as being composed basically of two components: (1) *body fat* and (2) *fat-free weight (lean body mass)*.

Component One — Body Fat

The amount of body fat (*adipose tissue*) that is stored is determined by two factors: (1) the number of fat-storing cells, or *adipocytes,* as they are called, and (2) the size, or capacity, of the adipocytes. The number of fat cells cannot be effectively decreased by exercise or dietary restrictions once adulthood is reached. During weight reduction involving fat loss in adults, it is the size but not the number of adipocytes that decreases. However, exercise and diet programs introduced during early childhood lead to a reduction in both the number and size of fat cells during the adult years. This is true even though the exercise and diet programs may not be continued into adulthood.

There is an old saying, "A fat baby is a healthy baby." From the standpoint of adulthood obesity, nothing could be farther from the truth. Overfeeding a child promotes increases in the number of his or her fat cells. If the fat cells are not subsequently decreased through exercise and diet programs during the childhood years, they cannot be decreased after adulthood is reached. Thus, the seed for obesity or overfatness has been planted.

In nonathletic college-age men, body fat accounts for approximately 15 percent of the total body weight; the corresponding figure for women is approximately 26 percent. Among athletes, regardless of sports preference, the body fat is generally lower, with the percentages again differing on the basis of sex. For example, male marathon runners are extremely lean, with body fat ranging between 1 and 9 percent of total body weight and averaging under 5 percent. Female long-distance runners are also exceptionally lean, but the lowest individual values are about 6 percent fat. The percent of body fat among various men and women athletes is given in Figure 6–1. Keep in mind that since athletes are low in body fat, their muscle mass is generally greater than that of their nonathletic counterparts.

At this point, it should be mentioned that recently there has been some concern that body fat values below 15 percent in women might be linked to menstrual irregularities, including *secondary amenorrhea* (the cessation of menstruation). This possibility, however, requires thorough scientific investigation and a good deal of further research. At the very least, the implications of such a possibility should be of concern to those familiar with the expert consensus that menstruation is not significantly affected (whatever the individual's percentage of body fat) by the activities associated with exercise and training. Clearly, in some women, the exact interrelationship of body fat, physical activity, and menstrual disorders remains to be determined.

Component Two — Fat-Free Weight (Lean Body Mass)

When the weight of body fat is subtracted from the total body weight, the remaining weight is referred to as *fat-free weight, lean body mass,* or *lean body weight.* The fat-free weight reflects mainly the skeletal muscle mass but also includes the weight of other tissues and organs such as bone and skin. The muscle mass makes up about 40 or 50 percent of the fat-free weight. The less body fat, the more fat-free weight. The average fat-free weight of college-age men is about 85 percent of their total body weight, and that of college-age women about 75 percent of their total body weight.

What is obesity or overfatness?

From the above discussion it should be apparent to you that obesity or overfatness refers to the above-average amount of fat contained in the body. This, in

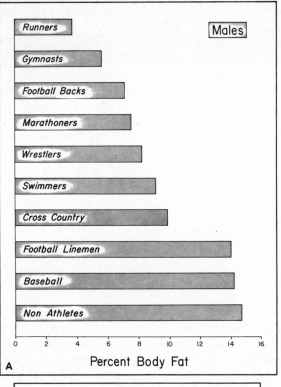

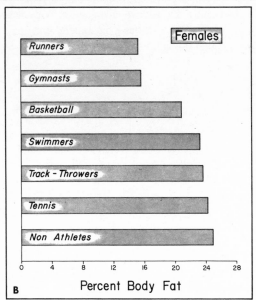

Figure 6–1. Percent body fat among various male athletes (A) and female athletes (B). The average body fat of college-age nonathletes is approximately 15 percent for males and 26 percent for females. Among athletes, regardless of sports preference, the body fat is generally lower for both sexes.

turn, is dependent upon the fat content of each fat cell and on the total number of fat cells present.

How do you know when you're obese or overfat? Probably the majority of us, if realistic, know whether or not we are overfat. Maybe we don't know by how much, but we know we're overfat! The best way to quantitate how overfat you are is to have your body composition assessed, that is, evaluate how much of your body is fat and how much is lean body mass or weight. You will learn how to estimate this in the next chapter. For now, you can use Table 6–1 as a guide to first, suggest whether you are overfat and, second, by how much. The body weights given in the table are based upon a sample of college-age men and women who, on the average, are not generally overfat. As a "rule of thumb," the majority of people will not be overfat if they weigh the same as they do, or did, when they are, or were, of college age (20 to 25 years old). A person whose weight is in excess of 25 percent of his or her college-age weight is considered to be obese (see Table 6–1).

CHANGING BODY WEIGHT

As mentioned in the last chapter, the maintenance of body weight is dependent upon a balance between energy (calories) taken in as food and energy (calories) expended to support bodily processes and physical activity. In other words, if you consume more calories than you expend, your body weight will increase. By the same token, if you expend more calories than you take in, body weight will decline. Therefore, in order to change your body weight, you need to know approximately how many calories you expend each day and how many calories you take in through the diet each day.

TABLE 6–1   Suggested Body Weights for Different Heights of College-Aged Men and Women*

| HEIGHT (inches) | BODY WEIGHT IN POUNDS | | | |
| | Men | | Women | |
	SUGGESTED	OBESE	SUGGESTED	OBESE
60			109	>136
62			115	>144
64	133	>166	122	>152
66	142	>177	129	>161
68	151	>189	136	>170
70	159	>199	144	>180
72	167	>209	152	>190
74	175	>219		
76	182	>228		

*Modified from Bogert, J., Briggs, G., and Calloway, D.: *Bogert's Nutrition and Physical Fitness,* 9th ed. Philadelphia: W. B. Saunders Co., 1973.

Estimating Your Caloric Expenditure

The number of calories you expend each day is based on your daily activity level. Your daily activity has two main parts: (1) a *basal* or *resting rate,* which accounts for the minimum activity of the body just in order to live; and, (2) a physical activity rate, which accounts for how active you are above the basal level. Both of these components are rather difficult to measure accurately. However, for our purposes, a reasonable estimate based on your body weight and physical activity level may be made from Table 6–2 for men and Table 6–3 for women. These tables have combined both parts of your daily activity. As an example, suppose you are a man and weigh 150 pounds (68 kilograms). Let's further suppose you are semiactive, that is, the amount of physical exercise you engage in daily is limited. From the table, your estimated energy expenditure over a 24-hour period would be roughly 2615 kilocalories. If you wanted to lose weight, your daily intake of calories would have to be less than 2615.

Estimating Your Caloric Intake

Counting the number of calories taken in through the diet means that you must record what kinds of food you've eaten and how much food or how many servings you've eaten during a 24-hour period. This is not an easy job, but when it is done, the number of calories taken in over a 24-hour day can be estimated with the help of Tables 6–4 and 6–5. Let's take an example. Suppose for breakfast you ate:

- 6 ounces (¾ cup) of orange juice
- 2 scrambled eggs
- 2 slices of whole wheat bread or toast
- 2 teaspoons of margarine
- 1 cup of regular instant coffee (black)

The number of kilocalories from Table 6–4 would be: 85 for the orange juice; 190 for the scrambled eggs; 130 (65 for each slice) for the bread or toast; 70 for the margarine; and 3 for the cup of coffee. This comes to a total of 478 kilocalories for breakfast. By doing this for each meal (and snacks too), the total number of calories eaten in 24 hours can be estimated. Note that the caloric values for fast foods are given in Table 6–5.

The above method of estimating your caloric intake is a difficult and tedious job. However, it is probably the most accurate method. There is another way to estimate your caloric intake, although it is less accurate than counting calories. It is based on your energy expenditure as estimated from Tables 6–2 and 6–3. The idea is that if your body weight is fairly constant* from week to week or month to month, your energy expenditure and energy intake are about the same. (*Text continued on page 94.*)

---

*Fairly constant means that your body weight fluctuates around two or three pounds per week. Remember, when comparing your body weight from week to week, weigh yourself at the same time of day each week.

TABLE 6–2 Suggested Energy Expenditures in Kilocalories for Different Body Weights and Activity Levels in Men

ACTIVITY LEVEL	BODY WEIGHT (MEN)											
	110 lb (50 kg)	120 lb (54 kg)	130 lb (59 kg)	140 lb (64 kg)	150 lb (68 kg)	160 lb (73 kg)	170 lb (77 kg)	180 lb (82 kg)	190 lb (86 kg)	200 lb (91 kg)	210 lb (95 kg)	220 lb (100 kg)
Sedentary Activity limited to routine sitting and walking	1680	1830	1985	2135	2288	2440	2595	2745	2900	3050	3205	3355
Semisedentary Activities involve standing and walking only	1800	1960	2125	2290	2450	2615	2780	2940	3105	3270	3430	3595
Semiactive Physically active but limited	1920	2090	2265	2440	2615	2790	2965	3140	3310	3485	3660	3835
Active Regular participation in sports activities or physical fitness programs	2040	2220	2410	2595	2780	2965	3150	3335	3520	3705	3890	4075
Very active Engaged in competitive sports or in vigorous daily fitness programs	2160	2355	2550	2745	2940	3140	3335	3530	3725	3920	4120	4315

TABLE 6–3   Suggested Energy Expenditures in Kilocalories for Different Body Weights and Activity Levels for Women

ACTIVITY LEVEL	BODY WEIGHT (WOMEN)										
	90 lb (41 kg)	100 lb (45 kg)	110 lb (50 kg)	120 lb (54 kg)	130 lb (59 kg)	140 lb (64 kg)	150 lb (68 kg)	160 lb (73 kg)	170 lb (77 kg)	180 lb (82 kg)
Sedentary Activity limited to routine sitting and walking	1235	1375	1510	1650	1790	1920	2060	2195	2335	2470
Semisedentary Activities involve standing and walking only	1325	1470	1620	1764	1915	2061	2205	2355	2500	2645
Semiactive Physically active but limited	1410	1570	1730	1880	2039	2195	2355	2510	2670	2825
Active Regular participation in sports activities or physical fitness programs	1500	1665	1835	2000	2170	2335	2500	2670	2835	3000
Very active Engaged in competitive sports or in vigorous daily fitness programs	1590	1765	1945	2120	2295	2470	2645	2825	3000	3175

TABLE 6-4　Caloric (Kilocalories) Values for Selected Foods*

Food	Weight gm	Approximate Measure	Energy Kcal
Almonds, chopped	15	12–15 nuts, 2 tbsp	90
Apples, raw with skin	150	1 medium 3/lb	80
Apple juice, canned, no sugar added	125	1/2 c	60
Applesauce, sweetened	125	1/2 c	120
Apricots			
Fresh	100	2–3 medium	50
Canned, heavy syrup	120	4 halves, 2 tbsp juice	100
water pack	100	4 halves, 2 tbsp juice	40
Dried, sulfured, raw	30	4–6 medium halves	80
Apricot nectar, canned	125	1/2 c	70
Artichokes, French, boiled	120	1 large (300 g as purchased)	30
Asparagus,²			
Fresh, green, cooked	100	1/2 c cut, 6–7 spears	20
Canned, salt added³	100	1/2 c cut, 6–7 spears	20
Avocados	125	1/2 fruit, 4 in long	190
Baby foods			
Dinners	130	Contents 4½ oz jar	
beef-noodle			60
beef-vegetable			110
vegetable-beef-cereal			70

Food	Weight gm	Approximate Measure	Energy Kcal
Beer	360	12 oz bottle	150
Beet greens, boiled	75	1/2 c	15
Beets, sliced, canned	85	1/2 c	30
Beverages. See Carbonated beverages, individual entries, a			
Biscuits, from mix, enriched	30	1 of 2 in diameter	90
Blackberries, boysenberries, etc., raw	70	1/2 c	40
Blueberries, raw	70	1/2 c	45
Bokchay. See Pakchoy.			
Brazil nuts, raw	30	6 large nuts	180
Bread			
Boston brown, canned	45	1 slice, ½ in thick	95
Corn, from mix	55	2½ in square	180
Cracked wheat	25	1 slice	65
French, Vienna, Italian, enriched	25	1 slice	70
Fry bread, Indian, enriched	60	1 piece, medium	200
Raisin, not enriched	25	1 slice	65
Rye, American	25	1 slice	65
White, not enriched enriched	25	1 slice	70
Whole-wheat	25	1 slice	65
Broccoli, fresh or frozen, boiled	85	1/2 c	20
Brussels sprouts, fresh or frozen, boiled	85	4 large sprouts	30

Food	Weight gm	Approximate Measure	Energy Kcal
Celery			
Raw	80	2 large stalks	15
Boiled	75	1/2 c diced	10
Cereals, breakfast			
Ready-to-eat			
bran flakes, 40% enr.	35	1 c	100
corn flakes, enriched	25	1 c	95
granola	50	1/2 c	215
rice, puffed, enriched	15	1 c	60
wheat flakes, enriched	30	1 c	100
wheat, shredded	50	1 c of spn-sized	180
Cooked, 1 oz. dry wt., salt added			
cornmeal and grits,			
unenriched	120	1/2 c	60
enriched	120	1/2 c	60
oatmeal	120	1/2 c	65
wheat, farina light, enriched (e.g., Cream of Wheat)	120	1/2 c	50
whole-meal (e.g., Ralston)	120	1/2 c	55
Chard, Swiss, boiled	70	1/2 c	15
Cheese			
Natural			
blue, Roquefort	30	1 oz	100
cheddar	30	1 oz	115
cottage, creamed	110	1/2 c	120
cream	30	2 tbsp	100
Parmesan	30	1 oz	130
Swiss	30	1 oz	110
Pasturized, processed			
American	30	1 oz	110
cheese spread	30	1 oz	80
Cheese fondue	100	2/3 c	260

Food	Weight (g)	Measure	Calories
Fruits and desserts		Contents 4¾ oz jar	
banana-pineapple	135		110
custard pudding			130
fruit pudding			130
Bacon, broiled, drained	25	2 strips, thick	140
Bagels	60	4 in diameter	180
Bamboo shoots	100	3/4 c	25
Bananas	120	1 medium	100
Beans			
Canned, with pork and tomato sauce	130	1/2 c	160
Canned, with pork and sweet sauce	130	1/2 c	190
Lima, fresh or frozen, boiled	85	1/2 c	95
Red, canned	125	1/2 c	120
Refried	120	1/2 c	230
Snap, green, fresh or frozen, boiled	65	1/2 c	15
canned	65	1/2 c	15
Soybeans, mature, dry, cooked	90	1/2 c (1 oz, dry wt.)	120
Bean sprouts. See Sprouts.			
Beef			
Corned, canned	80	2 slices each, 3 in x 2 in x ¼ in	170
hash, with potatoes	110	1/2 c	200
Dried, creamed	120	1/2 c	190
Hamburger, broiled, lean, 21% fat	85	4/lb, raw wt.	240
very lean, 10% fat	85	4/lb, raw wt.	190
Roast, chuck, braised	85	3 oz	240
rib, U.S. choice	85	3 oz	380
Steak, broiled			
round with fat	85	3 oz	220
sirloin with fat	85	3 oz	330
Beef stew, with vegetables	245	1 c	220

Food	Weight (g)	Measure	Calories
Butter, salted	5	1 tsp or pat (90/lb)	35
	15	1 tbsp	100
Cabbage, green, headed			
Raw, shredded	70	1 c	17
Cooked, chopped	70	1/2 c	15
Cakes			
Angel food	40	2 in sector of 10 in cake	105
Cheese cake, frozen[6]	85	1/10 of cake	225
Chocolate, with chocolate icing	90	2 in sector of 8 in cake	310
Gingerbread	65	2¾ in square	170
Cupcake, iced	50	1 medium	190
Pound cake	30	3½ in x 3 in x ½ in	140
Yellow with chocolate icing	70	2 in sector of 8 in cake	230
Candy			
Caramels	30	1 oz	120
Chocolate bar			
plain milk chocolate	30	1 oz	140
with almonds	30	1 oz	150
Fudge with nuts	30	1 oz	120
Hard	30	1 oz	110
Marshmallow	30	1 oz, 4 large	90
Peanut brittle	30	1 oz.	120
Cantaloupe. See Melons.			
Carbonated beverages sweet	170	6 oz	65
Carrots			
Raw	80	1 carrot, 7 1/2 in x 1 1/8 in	30
Boiled	70	1/2 c diced	20
Cashews, roasted	30	1 oz	160
Cauliflower			
Raw	50	1/2 c whole flower buds	15
Boiled	60	1/2 c	15

Food	Weight (g)	Measure	Calories
Cherries			
Raw, sweet	75	10 cherries	45
Red, canned			
heavy syrup	130	1/2 c with syrup	100
water pack	120	1/2 c with juice	50
Chicken			
Canned, flesh only	100	1/2 c	200
Creamed	120	1/2 c	210
Fried			
breast	95	1/2 breast	160
leg	55	1 medium	90
thigh	65	1 medium	120
Roasted, light meat, without skin	100	3½ oz	170
Chickpeas or garbanzos, cooked without salt	125	1/2 c (30 gm, dry wt.)	110
Chili con carne, with beans, canned	255	1 c	340
Chili powder, chilis. See Peppers.			
Chili relleno (stuffed pepper)	110	1 pepper	190
Chocolate, bitter or baking	30	1 oz	140
Sweet, milk. See Candy.			
Chow mein, canned, chicken without noodles	250	1 c	95
Clams, canned, with liquid	100	3½ oz, 1/2 c	50
Cocoa, dry	5	1 tbsp	15
Coconut, dry, unsweetened	30	1 oz	180
Coffee, instant, regular dry powder	2.5	1 tbsp	3
Collards, boiled	70	1/2 c	20

TABLE 6–4 Caloric (Kilocalories) Values for Selected Foods* (Continued)

Food	Weight gm	Approximate Measure	Energy Kcal
Cookies			
Commercial assortment	35	4 cookies	170
Fig bar	55	4 cookies	200
Oatmeal with raisins	50	4 cookies	235
Corn, sweet, yellow			
Fresh or frozen, boiled	80	1/2 c	70
Canned, whole kernel	80	1/2 c	70
Cream style	130	1/2 c	110
Corn fritter	35	1 fritter 2 in x 1½ in	130
Corn syrup	20	1 tbsp	60
Cowpeas or blackeye peas			
Immature	80	1/2 c	90
Mature, dry, cooked	125	1/2 c,(1oz dry wt.)	95
Crabmeat	100	1/2 c, packed	100
Crackers			
Butter (e.g., Ritz)	15	5 round	75
Graham	15	1 cracker 5 in x 2½ in	55
Rye wafer (e.g., Rykrisp)	15	2 wafers	40
Saltines	10	4 each, 2 in square	50
Cranberry jelly, or sauce, canned	35	1/8 c	50
Cream			
Half-and-half	60	1/4 c or 4 tbsp	80
Heavy, whipping	60	1/4 c; 1/2 c whipped vol	210
Light, for coffee	60	1/4 c, 4 tbsp	120
Sour	60	1/4 c, 4 tbsp	130

Food	Weight gm	Approximate Measure	Energy Kcal
Fish, Salmon (Continued)			
canned, pink	110	1/2 c	160
red	110	1/2 c	190
Sardines			
canned in oil	85	3 oz drained	170
Sole or flounder, fillet, baked	100	3 oz	200
Swordfish, broiled	100	3 oz	170
Tuna, raw	100	1/2 c	135
canned in oil	100	1/2 c	200
in water	100	1/2 c	130
Flour, wheat			
White, all purpose			
unenriched	115	1 c	420
enriched	115	1 c	420
Whole-grain	120	1 c	400
French toast, frozen[10]	65	1 slice	130
Frozen dinners			
Chicken, fried, with potatoes, mixed vegetables	310	11 oz dinner	570
Meat loaf with tomato sauce, potatoes, peas	310	11 oz dinner	410
Turkey with gravy, potatoes, peas	310	11 oz dinner	340
Fruit cocktail	130	1/2 c	95
Gelatin, dry	8	1 tbsp or packet	30
Gelatin dessert, plain	120	1/2 c	70
Grapefruit, raw	100	1/2 medium	40
Grapefruit juice, canned			
Unsweetened	180	3/4 c	75
Sweetened	180	3/4 c	100

Food	Weight gm	Approximate Measure	Energy Kcal
Lemonade, from frozen concentrate	250	1 c	110
Lentils, dried, cooked	100	1/2 c	110
Lettuce, raw			
Head, solid (iceberg type)	90	1/6 head	10
Loose leaf, romaine, cos	55	1 c, chopped	10
Liver			
Beef, fried	85	3 oz	200
Calf, fried	85	3 oz	220
Chicken, simmered	70	1/2 c, chopped	120
Lobster, northern, cooked	95	2/3 c meat	90
Lychee nuts, raw	150	10 nuts	60
Macaroni and other pastas, cooked			
Unenriched	130	1 c	190
Enriched	130	1 c	190
Macaroni with cheese, casserole, baked	200	1 c	430
Mangos, raw	165	1c, diced	110
Margarine	5	1 tsp, 1 pat (90/lb)	35
Melons			
Cantaloupe	160	1/2 melon or 1 c, cubed	50
Honeydew	170	1/8 melon or 1 c, cubed	55
Watermelon	425	1/16 melon (2lb with rind)	110

Food	g	Measure	Cal
Cream substitutes			
Coffee whitener	3	1 tsp or packet	15
Whipped topping, frozen	10	2 tbsp	30
Cucumber, raw, peeled	80	1/2 small	10
Custard, baked	130	1/2 c	150
Dandelion greens, boiled	50	1/2 c	20
Dasheen (Japanese taro), raw	100	1 1/3 corms	100
Dates, dried	80	10, pitted	220
Doughnuts			
Cake type	40	1 average	160
Yeast, raised	40	1 average	180
Eggnog	250	1 c	340
Eggs, chicken			
Whole, raw or hard cooked	50	1 large	80
white	33	1 white	15
yolk	17	1 yolk	65
Scrambled	140	2 eggs	190
Eggplant, boiled	100	1/2 c diced	20
Enchiladas, beef			
Frozen, commercial[10]	200	7 oz portion	240
Home recipe	190	2 enchiladas	365
Fats, shortening, solid	100	1/2 c	880
or oil	12	1 tbsp	110
Figs, fresh	100	2 medium	80
Dried	30	2 small	80
Fish			
Cod, steak, sautéed	110	4 oz	180
Fish sticks, breaded	110	4 sticks	200
Haddock, fried	110	4 oz	180
Mackerel, sautéed	105	3 average	250
Salmon, steak, broiled	145	1 average 6 in x 2 in	230
Grapes, raw			
Slip-skin	100	20 grapes	45
Adherent skin	100	20 grapes	70
Grape juice	190	3/4 c	120
Guacamole	120	1/2 c	140
Ham, baked	85	3 oz	250
Hominy grits. See *Cereal*, cooked.			
Honey, strained	20	1 tbsp	65
Ice cream, vanilla			
Plain, 10% fat	65	1/2 c	135
Rich, 16% fat	75	1/2 c	175
Ice milk, vanilla	65	1/2 c	90
Ices, water, lime	95	1/2 c	120
Jams and jellies	20	1 tbsp	55
Kale, boiled without stems	55	1/2 c	20
Kidney, braised	100	3 1/2 oz	250
Kohlrabi, boiled	80	1/2 c, diced	20
Kumquat, raw	20	1 medium	10
Lamb, choice grade			
Chop, loin, broiled			
lean and fat	95	1 average	340
lean only	65	1 average	120
Leg, roasted			
lean only	85	3 oz	160
Shoulder, roasted			
lean and fat	85	3 oz	280
Lard. See *Fats*.			
Lasagna, frozen[6]	225	8 oz serving	380
Lemon juice, fresh	15	1 tbsp	5
Milk, cow			
Whole, fluid	245	1 c	155
2%, low-fat	245	1 c	140
Skim, nonfat, or buttermilk	245	1 c	90
Chocolate, low-fat	250	1 c	180
Dried, instant			
whole	30	1/4 c	160
nonfat	35	1/4 c	125
Evaporated	250	1 c	340
Condensed, sweetened	40	1 fl oz	120
Milk, human, U.S.	30	1 fl oz	21
Milkshakes, commercial	270	10 fl oz	320
Molasses			
Light	20	1 tbsp	50
Medium	20	1 tbsp	50
Blackstrap	20	1 tbsp	45
Muffins			
Bran	40	1 muffin	100
Cornmeal	40	1 muffin	130
Plain or blueberry	40	1 muffin	120
Mushrooms, raw	35	1/2 c, sliced	10
Mustard greens, boiled	70	1/2 c	15
Mustard, prepared, yellow	5	1 tsp	4
Noodles, egg, cooked.			
Unenriched	105	2/3 c	130
Enriched	105	2/3 c	130
Oils. See *Fats*.			
Okra, boiled	105	10 pods	30
Olives			
Green	25	5 large	20
Ripe	25	5 large	35
Onions			
Green, raw, bulb and top	25	1/4 c, chopped or 3 onions	10
Mature, dry			
raw	85	1/2 c, chopped	30
	10	1 tbsp, 1/8 onion	4
boiled	105	1/2 c, sliced	30

TABLE 6–4   Caloric (Kilocalories) Values for Selected Foods* (*Continued*)

Food	Weight gm	Approximate Measure	Energy Kcal
Oranges, raw	140	1 medium	80
Orange juice, fresh or frozen	185	3/4 c	85
Oysters, raw			
Eastern	120	6 oysters	80
Pacific	120	6 oysters	110
Pakchoy, raw	100	2/3 c	15
Pancakes, plain	110	4, ea. 4 in diam.	245
Papaya, raw	225	1/2 fruit or 1 c, cubed	60
Parsley, raw	5	1 tbsp, chopped	2
Peaches, without skin			
Raw, yellow	115	1 medium	40
Canned, heavy syrup	150	2 halves and 3 tbsp juice	120
water pack	155	2 halves and 3 tbsp juice	50
Dried, sulfured, uncooked	65	5 halves	170
Peanuts, roasted, salted	30	1oz, 30 nuts	65
Peanut butter	15	1 tbsp	95
Pears			
Raw, with skin	180	1, 3½ x 2½ in	100
Canned, syrup	150	2 halves and 3 tbsp juice	115
water pack	155	2 halves and 3 tbsp juice	50
Peas			
Green, frozen, boiled	80	1/2 c	55

Food	Weight gm	Approximate Measure	Energy Kcal
Plantain	265	1 banana 11 in x 2 in	310
Plums, raw	70	1 medium	30
Canned, purple in heavy syrup	140	3 and 3 tbsp syrup	110
Popcorn with oil and salt	10	1 c	40
Pork			
Chop, broiled lean and fat	80	1 medium	300
lean only	50	1 medium	110
Loin, roasted lean and fat	85	2½ in x 2½ in x ¾ in	310
Spareribs, braised	90	yield from ½ lb, raw wt.	400
Potatoes			
Baked	200	1 large	140
Boiled, pared before cooking	135	1 medium	90
French-fried commercial[14] frozen, reheated	70	1 "order"	220
	100	20 strips	220
Mashed with milk	100	1/2 c	100
Potato chips	20	10 chips, 2 in diameter each	115
Potato salad. See *Salads.*			
Pretzels	30	10, 3-ring pretzels	120
Prunes, dried, raw	50	5	130
Cooked without sugar	125	1/2 c	120
Prune juice, canned	190	3/4 c	150

Food	Weight gm	Approximate Measure	Energy Kcal
Salad dressings (Continued)			
Salad dressing	15	1 tbsp	65
Thousand Island, or Louie-type	15	1 tbsp	80
Salmon. See *Fish.*			
Sandwiches			
Bacon, lettuce, tomato on white bread	150	1 average	280
Egg salad on white bread	140	1 average	280
Fish fillet, fried on bun[14]	135	1 average	410
Ham and cheese on white bread[15]	u	1 average	350
Hamburger on bun[14]	95	1 regular	250
"Big Mac"[14]	185	1 large	560
Tuna salad on white bread	105	1 average	280
Sashimi. See *Fish*, tuna, raw.			
Sardines. See *Fish.*			
Sauces			
Butterscotch	45	2 tbsp	200
Cheese	40	2 tbsp	65
Chocolate			
thin syrup	40	2 tbsp	100
fudge type	40	2 tbsp	125
Custard	70	1/4 c	85
Hard sauce	20	2 tbsp	95
Hollandaise	50	1/4 c scant	180
Soy	35	2 tbsp	25
Tartar	15	1 tbsp	75
Tomato catsup	15	1 tbsp	15
White, medium	125	1/2 c	200
Sauerkraut, canned	120	1/2 c	20

Food	g	Measure	Cal
Canned, drained	85	1/2 c	75
Split, dry, cooked	100	1/2 c (1 oz, dry wt.)	115
Peas and carrots, frozen, boiled	80	1/2 c	40
Pecans	30	1 oz, 20 halves	200.
Peppers, hot (chili)			
Green, canned sauce	15	1 tbsp	3
Red, dry, chili powder	3	1 tsp	8
Peppers, sweet			
Green, raw	75	1/2 c, chopped	15
Red, raw	90	1 medium	25
Pickles, cucumber			
Dill	135	1 large	15
Sweet	35	1 medium	50
Relish, sweet	15	1 tbsp	20
Pies			
Apple, berry, rhubarb	160	1/6 of 9 in pie	400
Cherry, peach	160	1/6 of 9 in pie	410
Cream, pudding type with meringue	150	1/6 of 9 in pie	380
Custard	150	1/6 of 9 in pie	330
Lemon meringue	140	1/6 of 9 in pie	360
Mince	160	1/6 of 9 in pie	430
Pecan	140	1/6 of 9 in pie	580
Pumpkin	150	1/6 of 9 in pie	320
Sweet potato	150	1/6 of 9 in pie	325
Pineapple, diced or crushed			
Raw	155	1 c	80
Canned, in heavy syrup	130	1/2 c solids and liquid	95
in juice	125	1/2 c solids and liquid	70
water pack	125	1/2 c solids and liquid	50
Pineapple juice	190	3/4 c	105
Pinenuts, piñon	30	1 oz, 4 tbsp	180
Pizza, cheese	65	1/8 of 14 in pizza	150
Sausage	65	1/8 of 14 in pizza	160

Food	g	Measure	Cal
Puddings			
Almendrado	65	1/3 c and 2 tbsp sauce	100
Apple Brown Betty	110	1/2 c	160
Capirotada	155	1/2 c	385
Chocolate, instant, packaged	130	1/2 c	160
Custard	130	1/2 c	150
Rice with raisins	130	1/2 c	200
Tapioca	80	1/2 c	110
Vanilla, home recipe	130	1/2 c	140
Pumpkin, canned	245	1 c	80
Radishes, raw	45	5 large	7
Raisins	35	1/4 c	100
Rhubarb, cooked with sugar	135	1/2 c	190
Rice cooked, salt added			
Brown	130	2/3 c	160
White, enriched	135	2/3 c	150
Precooked, instant	110	2/3 c	120
Rolls and buns			
Danish pastry	65	1, of 4 in diameter	270
Hamburger or frankfurter bun, enriched	40	1 average	120
Hard rolls, enriched	50	1 large	160
Plain pan rolls, white, enriched	30	1 small	85
Rutabagas, boiled	85	1/2 c, cubed	30
Salads			
Chef's (lettuce w/ham, cheese, dressing)[15]		1 serving	285
Potato, home recipe	125	1/2 c	120
Tuna fish	100	1/2 c	170
Salad dressings			
Blue cheese	15	1 tbsp	75
French, regular	15	1 tbsp	65
low-calorie	15	1 tbsp	15
Italian, regular	15	1 tbsp	85
low-calorie	15	1 tbsp	10
Mayonnaise	15	1 tbsp	100

Food	g	Measure	Cal
Sausages			
Bologna	30	1 slice, 4¼ in x 1/8 in	85
Frankfurter (all-meat)	45	1 average	135
Liverwurst	30	1 oz	85
Luncheon meat, pork, cured	30	1 oz	85
Pork sausage, links	40	3 links	185
Salami, dry	30	3 small slices	130
Vienna, canned	50	3 sausages	115
Scallops			
Breaded, fried	95	3½ oz	180
Steamed	95	3½ oz	105
Sesame seeds, hulled	40	1/4 c	220
Sherbet, orange	95	1/2 c	135
Shrimp, canned	85	3 oz	100
French-fried	85	3 oz	190
Soups			
Albondiga (meatballs in tomato broth)	240	1 c with 4 meatballs	340
Bean, with pork	250	1 c	170
Bouillon, broth, consomme	240	1 c	30
Cream soups, canned, diluted with water	240	1 c	65
diluted with milk	245	1 c	150
Chicken noodle, from dry mix	240	1 c	55
Clam chowder, Manhattan	245	1 c	80
Onion	240	1 c	35
Split pea	245	1 c	140
Tomato	245	1 c	90
Vegetable beef	245	1 c	80
Spaghetti			
Canned, with tomato sauce and meatballs[17]	210	1 can, 7½ oz	250
Home recipe, with tomato sauce			
with cheese	250	1 c	260
with meatballs	250	1 c	330
Spinach, fresh or frozen, boiled	90	1/2 c	20

TABLE 6–4 Caloric (Kilocalories) Values for Selected Foods* (Continued)

Food	Weight gm	Approximate Measure	Energy Kcal
Sprouts, raw			
Alfalfa	100	1 c, packed	40
Mung bean	100	1 c	35
Soybean	100	1 c	50
Squash			
Summer, boiled	90	1/2 c	10
Winter			
baked	100	1/2 c	65
boiled	120	1/2 c	45
Strawberries			
Fresh	100	2/3 c whole	35
Frozen, sweetened	170	2/3 c	160
Sugar			
Brown	220	1 c, packed	820
White			
granulated	200	1 c	770
	4	1 tsp	15
	8	1 tbsp	30
powdered			
Sunflower seeds, hulled	35	1/4 c	200
Sweet potatoes			
Baked in skin	145	1 potato, 5 in x 2 in	160
Boiled in skin	130	1/2 c mashed	150
Candied	105	1/2 c medium	180
Syrup, maple-flavored, artificial	20	1 tbsp	50
Tacos, beef	80	1 taco	160
Tamales canned	100	3½ oz	140
Home recipe, chicken	130	2 tamales	275

Food	Weight gm	Approximate Measure	Energy Kcal
Tea, instant	1	1/2 tsp	3
Tofu, soybean curd	120	1 piece, 2½ in x 2¾ in x 1 in	85
Tomatoes, raw	135	1 medium	25
Canned	120	1/2 c	25
Tomato juice, canned	180	3/4 c	35
Tomato paste	130	1/2 c	110
Tongue, beef, braised	100	3½ oz	250
Tortillas			
Corn, lime-treated	30	1, of 6 in diameter	65
White flour	30	1, of 6 in diameter	110
Tostada with beans and small portion of cheese	210	1 tostada	335
Tuna. See *Fish.*			
Turkey, roasted			
Light meat	85	2 slices, each 4 in x 2 in x ¼ in	150
Dark meat	85	4 slices, each 2½ in x 1½ in x ¼ in	170
Turnips, boiled	80	1/2 c, cubed	20
Turnip greens, boiled	70	1/2 c	15
Veal cutlet, broiled	85	3 oz	180

Food	Weight gm	Approximate Measure	Energy Kcal
Vinegar, cider	15	1 tbsp	2
Waffles			
Made from mix	75	1, of 7 in diameter	210
Frozen[18]	45	2 sections	120
Walnuts, English	100	1 c halves	650
	15	2 tbsp, chopped	100
Watercress, raw	35	10 sprigs	5
Wheat bran, crude	30	1 oz	60
Wheat germ, raw	30	1 oz	100
Toasted	30	1 oz	120
Wine, dessert (18.8%)	105	3½ fl oz	140
Table (12.2%)	100	3½ fl oz	85
Yeast			
Dry, active	5	1 tbsp	20
Brewer's, debittered	5	1 tbsp	25
Yogurt			
Low-fat			
plain	230	8 fl oz carton	145
fruit, sweetened	230	8 fl oz carton	225
Regular			
plain	230	8 fl oz carton	140

*Regular food values adapted from Briggs, G. M., and Calloway, D. H.: *Bogert's Nutrition and Physical Fitness*, 10th ed. Philadelphia: W. B. Saunders Co., 1979.

TABLE 6–5   Caloric (Kilocalories) Values for Fast Foods*

FAST FOODS	Wt (gm)	kcal	FAST FOODS	Wt (gm)	kcal
BURGER CHEF			**DAIRY QUEEN** (*Continued*)		
Big Shef	186	542	DQ Sandwich	60	140
Cheeseburger	104	304	Fiesta Sundae	269	570
Double Cheeseburger	145	434	Hot Fudge Brownie Delight	266	570
French Fries	68	187	Mr. Misty Float	404	440
Hamburger, Regular	91	258	Mr. Misty Freeze	411	500
Mariner Platter	373	680	**KENTUCKY FRIED CHICKEN**		
Rancher Platter	316	640	Individual Pieces		
Shake	305	326	(Original Recipe)		
Skipper's Treat	179	604	Drumstick	54	136
Super Shef	252	600	Keel	96	283
BURGER KING			Rib	82	241
Cheeseburger	–	305	Thigh	97	276
Hamburger	–	252	Wing	45	151
Whopper	–	606	9 Pieces	652	1892
French Fries	–	214	**LONG JOHN SILVER'S**		
Vanilla Shake	–	332	Breaded Oysters, 6 pc	–	460
Whaler	–	486	Breaded Clams, 5 oz	–	465
Hot Dog	–	291	Chicken Planks, 4 pc	–	458
DAIRY QUEEN			Cole Slaw, 4 oz	–	138
Big Brazier Deluxe	213	470	Corn on Cob, 1 pc	–	174
Big Brazier Regular	184	457	Fish w/Batter, 2 pc	–	318
Big Brazier w/Cheese	213	553	Fish w/Batter, 3 pc	–	477
Brazier w/Cheese	121	318	Fryes, 3 oz	–	275
Brazier Cheese Dog	113	330	Hush Puppies, 3 pc	–	153
Brazier Chili Dog	128	330	Ocean Scallops, 6 pc	–	257
Brazier Dog	99	273	Peg Leg w/Batter, 5 pc	–	514
Brazier French Fries, 2.5 oz	71	200	Shrimp w/Batter, 6 pc	–	269
Brazier French Fries, 4.0 oz	113	320	Treasure Chest		
Brazier Onion Rings	85	300	2 pc Fish, 2 Peg Legs	–	467
Brazier Regular	106	260	**McDONALD'S**		
Fish Sandwich	170	400	Egg McMuffin	132	352
Fish Sandwich w/Cheese	177	440	English Muffin, Buttered	62	186
Super Brazier	298	783	Hot Cakes, w/Butter & Syrup	206	472
Super Brazier Dog	182	518	Sausage (Pork)	48	184
Super Brazier Dog w/Cheese	203	593	Scrambled Eggs	77	162
Super Brazier Chili Dog	210	555	Big Mac	187	541
Banana Split	383	540	Cheeseburger	114	306
Buster Bar	149	390	Filet O Fish	131	402
DQ Choc Dipped Cone, sm	78	150	French Fries	69	211
DQ Choc Dipped Cone, med	156	300	Hamburger	99	257
DQ Choc Dipped Cone, lg	234	450	Quarter Pounder	164	418
DQ Chocolate Malt, sm	241	340	Quarter Pounder w/Cheese	193	518
DQ Chocolate Malt, med	418	600	Apple Pie	91	300
DQ Chocolate Malt, lg	588	840	Cherry Pie	92	298
DQ Chocolate Sundae, sm	106	170	McDonaldland Cookies	63	294
DQ Chocolate Sundae, med	184	300	Chocolate Shake	289	364
DQ Chocolate Sundae, lg	248	400	Strawberry Shake	293	345
DQ Cone, sm	71	110	Vanilla Shake	289	323
DQ Cone, med	142	230	**PIZZA HUT**		
DQ Cone, lg	213	340	Thin 'N Crispy†		
Dairy Queen Parfait	284	460	Beef†	–	490
Dilly Bar	85	240	Pork†	–	520
DQ Float	397	330	(*Continued on next page*)		
DQ Freeze	397	520			

TABLE 6–5 Caloric (Kilocalories) Values for Fast Foods* (*Continued*)

FAST FOODS	Wt (gm)	kcal	FAST FOODS	Wt (gm)	kcal
PIZZA HUT (*Continued*)			TACO BELL (*Continued*)		
Cheese	–	450	Taco	83	186
Pepperoni	–	430	Tostada	138	179
Supreme	–	510	BEVERAGES		
Thick 'N Chewy†			Coffee, 6 oz	180	2
Beef‡	–	620	Tea, 6 oz	180	2
Pork‡	–	640	Orange Juice, 6 oz	183	82
Cheese	–	560	Chocolate Milk, 8 oz	250	213
Pepperoni	–	560	Skim Milk, 8 oz	245	88
Supreme	–	640	Whole Milk, 8 oz	244	159
TACO BELL			Coca-Cola, 8 oz	246	96
Bean Burrito	166	343	Fanta Ginger Ale, 8 oz	244	84
Beef Burrito	184	466	Fanta Grape, 8 oz	247	114
Beefy Tostada	184	291	Fanta Orange, 8 oz	248	117
Bellbeefer	123	221	Fanta Root Beer, 8 oz	246	103
Bellbeefer w/Cheese	137	278	Mr. Pibb, 8 oz	245	93
Burrito Supreme	225	457	Mr. Pibb Without Sugar, 8 oz	237	1
Combination Burrito	175	404	Sprite, 8 oz	245	95
Enchirito	207	454	Sprite Without Sugar, 8 oz	237	3
Pintos 'N Cheese	158	168	Tab, 8 oz	237	tr
			Fresca, 8 oz	237	2

Note: Fast foods tend to be:
1. high in calories;
2. low in vitamin A;
3. low in fiber;
4. high in sodium;
5. adequate in protein;
6. high in cost compared to a comparable product made at home.

*Adapted from Young, E. A., Brennan, E. H., and Irving, G. L. (guest eds.): "Perspectives on fast foods." *Public Health Currents* 19(1), 1970, published by Ross Laboratories, Columbus, OH 43216.

†Based on a serving size of ½ of a 10-inch pizza (3 slices).

‡Topping mixture of ingredient.

Therefore, under these conditions, and these conditions only, your energy expenditure is a good estimate of your energy intake through the diet.

Once the number of calories expended through activity and the number of calories taken in through the diet are known, you are ready to either lose fat or gain muscle mass or lean body weight.

Losing Body Fat

In order to lose body fat, more calories need to be expended than are taken in. Actually, it requires an excess expenditure of 3500 calories in order to lose one pound of pure fat. If that sounds like a lot of calories for just one pound, it is! This is one of the reasons why a *diet program* combined with an *exercise program* is the most effective way to lose weight. For example, when dieting, you decrease the number of calories taken in and, when exercising, you increase the number of calories expended, thus maximizing the difference between caloric expenditure and caloric intake (referred to as the caloric deficit).

Another reason why both diet and exercise programs are most effective in losing body weight is that together they promote fat loss while preserving lean body weight. In other words, more fat and less muscle are lost when exercise and diet programs are combined. With diet alone, even with the same caloric deficit, greater amounts of muscle mass are lost.

Let's take a specific example of how diet and exercise programs work together in promoting body fat loss. Suppose you are a sedentary woman who weighs 150 pounds but needs to lose 20 pounds. Referring to Table 6-3, your caloric expenditure would be approximately 2060 kilocalories. Assuming that your body weight has been steady at 150 pounds for the past few weeks or so, your caloric intake would also be roughly 2060 kilocalories. Now suppose you begin regular exercise programs of lifting weights three days per week and walking and jogging five days per week. At the same time, you diet (seven days per week), dropping from your usual 2060 kilocalories intake to 1400 kilocalories. (A 1400 kilocalories diet is given in Table 5-4, p. 75). How much weight will you lose per week and how long will it take you to lose 20 pounds?

Your physical activity level will increase from 2060 kilocalories to about 2500 as your exercise programs have now increased your activity level from sedentary to active. At the same time, your diet will reduce your caloric intake to 1400 kilocalories. The caloric deficit for five days per week will be (2500 – 1400) × 5 = 5500 kilocalories. On two days a week, you do not exercise but your caloric deficit due to your diet will be (2060 – 1400) × 2 = 1320 kilocalories. The total deficit for the week will then be 5500 + 1320 kilocalories = 6820 kilocalories. Since it requires an excess expenditure of 3500 kilocalories to lose one pound of pure fat, you should lose 6820 ÷ 3500 = 1.9 or approximately 2.0 pounds per week. It will take you 10 weeks to reach your weight-loss goal of 20 pounds.

Let's take another example. This time suppose you are a man who weighs 190 pounds but who needs to lose 40 pounds. Again, let's say that you are sedentary. Referring to Table 6-2, if you are maintaining your body weight steady at 190 pounds, then your caloric intake and expenditure are the same or approximately 2900 kilocalories. Starting your five-day per week exercise program brings your caloric expenditure up to 3520 kilocalories. A diet of 1400 kilocalories would be too low for this high expenditure level. Therefore, you will need to use a 2000 kilocalories diet. (Such a diet is shown in Table 6-6.) For five days, the caloric deficit will then be (3520 – 2000) × 5 = 7600 kilocalories. Your two-day caloric deficit while continuing to diet but not exercising will be (2900 – 2000) × 2 = 1800. The total deficit for the week will be 7600 + 1800 = 9400 kilocalories. This means that 9400 ÷ 3500 = 2.7 pounds of weight will be lost per week, requiring about 15 weeks to lose 40 pounds.

The above examples are for adults. Weight-loss programs for children are essentially the same with the exception that dietary restrictions should not fall under 2000 kilocalories per day, particularly for young boys. Levels less than this may compromise growth. As mentioned previously, a 2000 kilocalorie diet is given in Table 6–6.

Water loss versus fat loss

Don't be fooled by the claims of many health spas that you can lose up to "25 inches or 14 pounds in just three days!" While such claims may be true, the loss of weight is mainly water, not fat. Of course, this kind of weight loss is neither permanent nor does it significantly affect your body composition. In fact, if continued for prolonged periods of time, it can even be dangerous. As has been emphasized throughout this chapter, loss of body fat is a *slow* process.

TABLE 6–6   Example of a Low-Calorie (2000-kcal) Diet in Five Meals*

Breakfast	Snack
½ cup orange juice	1 banana
1 soft-boiled egg	
1 slice whole wheat toast	Total kilocalories: 100
2 teasp. margarine	
1 glass skim milk or other beverage	
Total kilocalories: 345	

Lunch	Snack
1 hamburger (3 oz) on a roll with relish	1 carton fruit-flavored yogurt
½ sliced tomato	1 cup grape juice
1 glass skim milk	
1 medium apple	Total kilocalories: 385
Total kilocalories: 510	

Dinner

1 serving of baked chicken marengo (½ breast)
¾ cup rice
5–6 brussel sprouts
1 bowl of green salad with French dressing
1 small piece gingerbread
1 cup skim milk or other beverage

Total kilocalories: 660

Daily total kilocalories: 2000

*From Smith, N. J.: *Food for Sport*, Palo Alto, California: Bull Publishing Co., 1976.

Spot reducing

Many people believe that by exercising a specific body area (or spot), the fat stored in that area will be selectively reduced. That is not true. Research has shown that regardless of what area is exercised, the fat stores are reduced all over the body, not just selectively from one area. Therefore, spot reducing is a myth.

Tips on starting your weight (fat) loss program

The following guidelines should be helpful in achieving your weight (fat) loss goals:

- *First,* remember that it requires an excess expenditure of 3500 kilocalories in order to lose one pound of pure fat.
- *Second,* it is recommended that for adults the caloric deficit not exceed 2000 to 2500 kilocalories per day or an absolute maximum of four pounds of fat loss per week. An ideal loss is between two and three pounds per week. An attempt to estimate daily or weekly caloric intake and expenditure should be made. This may be done with the help of Tables 6–2, 6–3, 6–4, and 6–5.
- *Third,* the caloric deficit (the difference between calories taken in and calories expended) should represent both an increased caloric expenditure through exercise programs and a reduced caloric intake through dietary restrictions. A caloric deficit that is solely the result of dietary restrictions will cause loss of muscle mass or lean body weight.
- *Fourth,* dietary restrictions should not fall under 2000 kilocalories per day for young boys and girls. Levels less than this may compromise growth.
- *Fifth,* stick with it! Remember, it's going to take several months or longer to lose 20 pounds or more. You probably didn't get overfat overnight, therefore, don't expect to become lean again overnight!

Gaining Muscle Mass (Lean Body Weight)

For most people, gaining weight is easy. Unfortunately, the gain is mostly in body fat, which, as repeatedly emphasized, can lead to health problems. Ideally, increases in weight should reflect gains in muscle mass or lean body weight. Such gains are often desired by athletes, since lean body weight is generally positively correlated with athletic performance.

As you know by now, in order to gain weight your caloric intake must be greater than your caloric expenditure. It requires an excess intake of 2500 kilocalories in order to gain one pound of fat-free weight (muscle mass). To ensure that the excess calories will be laid down primarily as muscle mass and not fat, exercise programs such as those described in Chapters 3 and 4 should be undertaken.

The following is an example of how to gain fat-free weight by combining diet and exercise programs.

Suppose you are a 200-pound football player who wants to gain 25 pounds of muscle mass for the upcoming season. You should start your training programs that involve repeated 40-, 50-, and 100-yard sprints three days per week (Monday, Wednesday, and Friday), and also a weight training program three days per week (Tuesday, Thursday, and Saturday). From Table 6-3, your caloric expenditure should be roughly 3920 kilocalories per day (your training programs are vigorous and therefore classify you as very active). Your daily dietary intake can be increased to 5000 kilocalories. (Such a diet is given in Table 6-7.) With a dietary

TABLE 6-7   Example of a High-Calorie (5000-kcal) Diet in Five Meals*

Breakfast

½ cup orange juice
1 cup oatmeal
1 cup low-fat milk
1 scrambled egg
1 slice whole wheat toast
1½ teasp. margarine
1 tablespoon jam

Total kilocalories: 665

Snack

1 peanut butter sandwich
1 banana
1 cup grape juice

Total kilocalories: 485

Lunch

5 fish sticks with tartar sauce
1 large serving, French fries
1 bowl of green salad with avocado
    and French dressing
1 cup lemon sherbet
2 granola cookies
1 cup low-fat milk

Total kilocalories: 1505

Snack

1 cup mixed dried fruit
1½ cup malted milk

Total kilocalories: 660

Dinner

1 cup cream of mushroom soup
2 pieces oven-baked chicken
1 candied sweet potato
1 dinner roll and margarine
1 cup carrots and peas
½ cup cole slaw
1 piece cherry pie
1 beverage

Total kilocalories: 1615

Daily total kilocalories: 4930

*Modified from Smith, N. J.: *Food for Sport*, Palo Alto, California: Bull Publishing Co., 1976.

intake of 5000 kilocalories and an energy expenditure of 3920 kilocalories, there will be a daily excess intake of 1080 kilocalories, or for a six-day week, 6480 kilocalories. Since it requires an excess of 2500 kilocalories to gain one pound of muscle, it will take you 10 weeks or 2½ months in order to gain 25 pounds of lean body weight. Like fat loss, the gain in lean body weight is also *slow*.

Tips on starting your weight (muscle mass) gain program

Here are some guidelines to follow in starting your weight gain program.

- *First,* remember, in order to gain one pound of fat-free weight (muscle), an excess intake of 2500 kilocalories is required. An excess of this size should *not* be taken in one day.
- *Second,* it is recommended that the daily caloric intake not exceed expenditure by more than 1000 to 1500 kilocalories. On the basis of five diet days per week, this would mean a gain of 2 to 3 pounds per week.
- *Third,* an estimate of how many calories are being taken in and how many are being expended daily or weekly should be made. As mentioned previously, this can be done with the help of Tables 6–2, 6–3, 6–4, and 6–5.
- *Fourth,* to ensure that the excess calories will be laid down primarily as muscle and not fat, exercise training programs of the kind outlined in Chapters 3 and 4 should be adopted.
- *Fifth,* as with fat loss, the gain in lean body weight is a slow process. Set your weight gain goals according to the principles outlined here and stick with it.

7 □ Appraising Your Fitness Programs

How do you know that your fitness programs are improving your fitness levels? There are two answers to this question. The first one involves your overall feelings. For example, just as you can tell when you have overeaten, so will you be able to gauge, in very general terms, your physical fitness level. Indeed, the feeling of well being that comes from properly prescribed fitness programs is so strong that it will eventually become your principal motivator for continuing with your exercises. Futhermore, if you have to stop your fitness programs temporarily because of injury or illness, the desire to achieve, once again, that feeling of fitness will be a powerful motivator in your recovery.

The second answer involves the results derived from specific fitness tests. Describing these tests and interpreting their results will be the major purpose of this chapter. Primarily, we will deal with the progress you have made from the beginning of your fitness programs. Like your feelings, evaluation and actual measurement of your progress will help you in maintaining both interest and motivation in your fitness programs. Good evaluation will also help you to adjust your fitness programs so the most beneficial results can be obtained.

Your appraisal program should consist of tests selected to evaluate (1) your heart-lung system or endurance fitness program; (2) your muscular fitness program or, more specifically, your muscular strength, muscular endurance, and flexibility; and (3) your nutritional fitness program, including body composition changes.

MEDICAL EXAMINATION

Actually, your evaluation program starts with your prefitness program medical examination. As mentioned in Chapter 3 (p. 32), no one should begin an exercise fitness program without first obtaining a physician's approval. In addition to the physical examination, your physician may wish to conduct an exercise "stress test." Such a test usually involves recording your heart rate, blood pressure, and the results of an electrocardiogram,* and sometimes how much oxygen you are consuming while seated and standing and during and following exercise.

The exercise for the stress test can consist of either walking or jogging on a motor-driven treadmill (see Figure 7–1), or pedaling a stationary bicycle or even stepping up and down on a bench. Regardless of the mode of exercise used for the stress test, the intensity of the exercise is graduated so that light loads are used at the beginning of the test, with progressively harder and harder loads used by the end of the test. This kind of test primarily aids in the clinical assessment of your heart-lung or cardiorespiratory system. Whether or not you should have a stress test before starting your fitness program is up to the discretion of your personal physician.

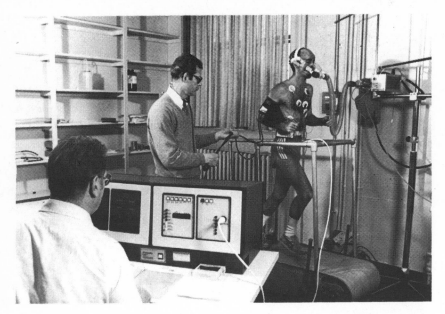

Figure 7–1. A stress test performed on a motor-driven treadmill. The electrodes on the runner's chest allow the electrical activity of the heart muscle to be recorded on the machine in the foreground (electrocardiogram). The cuff around the runner's upper right arm is used to measure blood pressure. The mouthpiece and attached tubing allow for measurement of the runner's maximal oxygen consumption. (Photo by Doug Martin, The Ohio State University Public Affairs Office.)

---

*An electrocardiogram is a tracing of the electrical activity of the heart muscle.

EVALUATION OF YOUR ENDURANCE FITNESS LEVEL

There are several ways in which you can evaluate your endurance fitness level. Regardless of which test you use, the test should be performed at the beginning of your program and then again after 8 to 10 weeks of training.

The Maximal Oxygen Consumption Test

The best way to evaluate endurance fitness is through a test called the *maximal oxygen consumption test*. Maximal oxygen consumption refers to how much oxygen you can take in or consume in one minute while you are performing maximal exercise. You will recall that endurance fitness is defined as the capacity or ability of the heart-lung system to deliver blood and thus oxygen to the working muscles during prolonged physical exercise. Therefore, measuring how much oxygen is consumed reflects how much is being delivered to the working muscles.

Unfortunately, the maximal oxygen consumption test is very difficult not only for the person taking the test but also for those who are administering the test. In the first case, the person taking the test is asked to exercise until he or she is exhausted. This, of course, demands a lot of effort and, in some cases, is very uncomfortable. Also, such a test usually costs a lot of money! In the second case, a lot of expensive equipment and highly trained technicians are required to perform the test (see Figure 7–1). It is also a good idea for a physician to be present when you take the test. So, all in all, while the test is an excellent indicator of your heart-lung function and your level of endurance fitness, it is, for most of you, impractical to use routinely to evaluate your endurance program.

The Resting Heart Rate Test

In Chapter 3, it was mentioned that endurance training programs cause an increased circulatory efficiency. This means that, after training, the heart pumps a certain amount of blood with a lower heart rate and a higher stroke volume than before training. In other words, one of the first signs of improvement in your heart-lung function is a decrease in your heart rate. Therefore, one of the ways in which you can evaluate the effects of your endurance fitness program is by comparing your resting heart rate before and after you started your endurance program. If your program increased your endurance fitness level, then your resting heart rate should be lower after training.

It is a good idea, then, for evaluation purposes, to keep a record of your resting heart rate from week to week. To do this, you should take your resting rate at the same time of the day. The best time is in the morning when you are awake but before you're out of bed. As mentioned previously (p. 32), your resting heart rate can be easily determined by palpation at any of several arteries (e.g., at the wrist, the neck, or the temple).

The Exercise Heart Rate Test

If possible, it also is a good idea to keep a record of your heart rate response when you're performing a given amount of light or moderate exercise. To do this, however, requires some sort of an ergometer (*ergo* = work, *meter* = measure) in order to precisely control the exercise load. Suitable ergometers are stationary bicycles, motor-driven treadmills, and step benches. The important point here is to make certain that each time you take the exercise heart rate test you are performing the same amount of exercise. If you use a bicycle ergometer, the pedaling rate and the resistance against which you pedal should be the same each time. If you use a treadmill, both the speed of the treadmill and its elevation should be the same for each test. For the step bench, the height of the bench and the stepping frequency should be kept constant from test to test. Regardless of which ergometer you use, keep the exercise light, that is, only hard enough to raise your heart rate to about 60 percent target heart rate level (see p. 32). The total duration of the exercise should be only 4 or 5 minutes.

Also, remember that it is not possible to accurately take your pulse rate while you are exercising. However, the pulse count obtained in a 6- or 10-second span immediately following exercise is a reasonable indicator of what your heart rate was during exercise. A 6-second count would be multiplied by 10 and a 10-second count by 6 in order to convert to beats per minute (see Table 7–1).

An example of records of both your resting and exercise heart rates during your endurance training program is given in Table 7–2.

Bench Step Test (Recovery Heart Rate Test)

The heart rate can be used in yet another way to evaluate your endurance fitness level. This involves taking your pulse rate after you have performed a given amount of exercise (referred to as the recovery heart rate). The most popular recovery heart rate tests are the Harvard Step Test for men and the Sloan Test for women.

For the step tests you'll need a bench or a firm chair or stool that is 20 inches high for men or 17 inches high for women. As shown in Figure 7–2, step up with both feet onto the bench, one foot at a time, then back down at a rate of 30 steps per minute* for as long as you can or up to 5 minutes. Take your pulse

---

*To keep the stepping cadence, you may use a stopwatch, a wall clock with a sweep second hand, or, better yet, a metronome (like musicians use to mark time).

TABLE 7–1 Conversion of 6- and 10-Second Pulse Counts
to Heart Rate in Beats per Minute

6-SECOND PULSE COUNT	HEART RATE (beats/minute)	10-SECOND PULSE COUNT	HEART RATE (beats/minute)
6	60	10	60
7	70	11	66
8	80	12	72
9	90	13	78
10	100	14	84
11	110	15	90
12	120	16	96
13	130	17	102
14	140	18	108
15	150	19	114
16	160	20	120
17	170	21	126
18	180	22	132
19	190	23	138
20	200	24	144
		25	150
		26	156
		27	162
		28	168
		29	174
		30	180
		31	186
		32	192
		33	198

from 1 to 1½ minutes after stopping (count for the entire 30-second period). Your fitness index is calculated by the following formula:

$$\text{Fitness Index} = \frac{(\text{Duration of exercise in seconds}) \times 100}{5.5 \times (\text{Pulse count from 1 to 1½ minutes after exercise})}$$

TABLE 7–2 An Example Record of Resting and Exercise Heart Rates
during an Endurance Training Program

DATE	RESTING HEART RATE (beats/minute)	EXERCISE* HEART RATE (beats/minute)
January 6 (start program)	78	148
January 20	75	145
February 1	72	144
February 15	70	142
March 1	66	139
March 15	63	135
March 29	59	130

*Exercise performed at a standard load during each test.

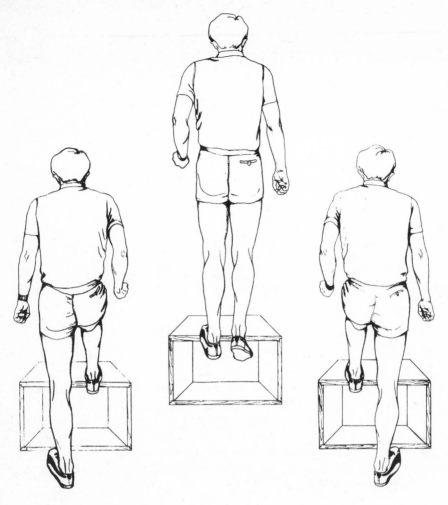

Figure 7-2. The Bench Step Test for evaluation of end..rance fitness. Step up with both feet onto the bench, one foot at a time, and then step back down at a rate of 30 steps per minute for as long as you can or for up to 5 minutes.

As an example, suppose you are a 25-year-old woman who exercised the full 5 minutes (300 seconds) and whose 1- to 1½-minute postexercise pulse count is 72 beats. Your fitness index or score would be 75. If you don't like to use a formula, you may use Table 7-3 for determining your fitness index.

Standards for interpreting your score are contained in Table 7-4 for men and Table 7-5 for women. The 25-year-old woman from the above example with a fitness index of 75 would have an average level of endurance fitness (Table 7-5).

TABLE 7–3　Scoring Table for Harvard Step Test and Sloan Test

DURATION OF TEST	HEART BEATS FROM 1 TO 1½ MINUTES IN RECOVERY										
	40–44	45–49	50–54	55–59	60–64	65–69	70–74	75–79	80–84	85–89	90–over
0 – 29"	5	5	5	5	5	5	5	5	5	5	5
0' 30"–0' 59"	20	15	15	15	15	10	10	10	10	10	10
1' 0"–1' 29"	30	30	25	25	20	20	20	20	15	15	15
1' 30"–1' 59"	45	40	40	35	30	30	25	25	25	20	20
2' 0"–2' 29"	60	50	45	45	40	35	35	30	30	30	25
2' 30"–2' 59"	70	65	60	55	50	45	40	40	35	35	35
3' 0"–3' 29"	85	75	70	60	55	55	50	45	45	40	40
3' 30"–3' 59"	100	85	80	70	65	60	55	55	50	45	45
4' 0"–4' 29"	100	100	90	80	75	70	65	60	55	55	50
4' 30"–4' 59"	125	110	100	90	85	75	70	65	60	60	55
5'	130	115	105	95	90	80	75	70	65	65	60

Cooper's 12-Minute Test

A fairly easy test to use to evaluate your endurance fitness (but not necessarily easy to perform) is Cooper's 12-Minute Test. The test involves walking and/or running as far as you can in 12-minutes. It's easy to use since it only requires a track (e.g., a quarter-mile track around a high school football field) and a stopwatch. The test can also be performed by swimming or cycling. Tables 7–6 (men) and 7–7 (women) contain standards for walking/running, swimming, and cycling distances along with their respective endurance fitness classifications.

TABLE 7–4　Standards for the Harvard Step Test (Men)*

FITNESS INDEX	AGE GROUPS (YEARS)		
	Under 30	30–50	Over 50
Under 54	Poor	Poor	Poor
54–67	Fair	Average	Good
68–82	Average	Good	Excellent
83–96	Good	Excellent	
Over 96	Excellent		

*Based on data from Fox, E. L., Billings, C. E., Bartels, R. L., Bason, R., and Mathews, D.: Fitness standards for male college students. Int. Z. angew. Physiol. 31:231–236, 1973.

TABLE 7–5   Standards for the Sloan Test (Women)*

| FITNESS INDEX | AGE GROUPS (YEARS) | | |
	Under 30	30–50	Over 50
Under 55	Poor	Poor	Poor
55–67	Fair	Average	Good
68–79	Average	Good	Excellent
80–90	Good	Excellent	
Over 90	Excellent		

*Based on data from Sloan, A. W.: A modified Harvard Step Test for women. *J. Appl. Physiol.* **14**:985–986, 1959.

TABLE 7–6   Guidelines for Cooper's 12-Minute Test for Running, Swimming, and Cycling for Men*

| CLASSIFI-CATION | RUNNING Age Groups (years) | | | |
	Under 30	30–39	40–49	50 and up
Very poor	Under 1.0 mile	Under .95 mile	Under .85 mile	Under .80 mile
Poor	1.0–1.24	.95–1.14	.85–1.04	.80–.99
Fair	1.25–1.49	1.15–1.39	1.05–1.29	1.0–1.24
Good	1.50–1.74	1.40–1.64	1.30–1.54	1.25–1.49
Excellent	Over 1.74	Over 1.64	Over 1.54	Over 1.49

| CLASSIFI-CATION | SWIMMING Age Groups (years) | | | |
	Under 30	30–39	40–49	50 and up
Very poor	Under 440 yards	Under 418 yards	Under 374 yards	Under 352 yards
Poor	440–545	418–502	374–458	352–435
Fair	546–655	503–612	459–568	436–545
Good	656–765	613–722	569–678	546–655
Excellent	Over 765	Over 722	Over 678	Over 655

| CLASSIFI-CATION | CYCLING Age Groups (years) | | | |
	Under 30	30–39	40–49	50 and up
Very poor	Under 2.50 miles	Under 2.38 miles	Under 2.12 miles	Under 2.00 miles
Poor	2.5–3.10	2.38–2.85	2.12–2.60	2.00–2.47
Fair	3.11–3.72	2.86–3.47	2.61–3.22	2.48–3.10
Good	3.73–4.35	3.48–4.10	3.23–3.85	3.11–3.72
Excellent	Over 4.36	Over 4.10	Over 3.85	Over 3.72

*Running distances are based on data from Cooper, K.: *The New Aerobics.* New York: M. Evans Co., 1970, p. 30. Swimming distances were calculated by dividing the running distances by 4; cycling distances, by multiplying the running distances by 2.5.

TABLE 7-7 Guidelines for Cooper's 12-Minute Test for Running, Swimming, and Cycling for Women*

CLASSIFI-CATION	RUNNING Age Groups (years)			
	Under 30	30–39	40–49	50 and up
Very poor	Under .95 mile	Under .85 mile	Under .75 mile	Under .65 mile
Poor	.95–1.14	.85–1.04	.75–.94	.65–.84
Fair	1.15–1.34	1.05–1.24	.95–1.14	.85–1.04
Good	1.35–1.64	1.25–1.54	1.15–1.44	1.05–1.34
Excellent	Over 1.64	Over 1.54	Over 1.44	Over 1.34

CLASSIFI-CATION	SWIMMING Age Groups (years)			
	Under 30	30–39	40–49	50 and up
Very poor	Under 418 yards	Under 374 yards	Under 330 yards	Under 286 yards
Poor	418–502	374–458	330–414	287–370
Fair	503–612	459–568	415–502	371–458
Good	613–722	569–678	503–634	459–590
Excellent	Over 722	Over 678	Over 634	Over 590

CLASSIFI-CATION	CYCLING Age Groups (years)			
	Under 30	30–39	40–49	50 and up
Very poor	Under 2.37 miles	Under 2.12 miles	Under 1.87 miles	Under 1.62 miles
Poor	2.37–2.85	2.12–2.60	1.87–2.35	1.62–2.10
Fair	2.86–3.35	2.61–3.10	2.36–2.85	2.11–2.60
Good	3.36–4.10	3.11–3.85	2.86–3.60	2.61–3.35
Excellent	Over 4.10	Over 3.85	Over 3.60	Over 3.35

*Running distances are based on data from Cooper, K.: *The New Aerobics.* New York: M. Evans Co., 1970, p. 30. Swimming distances were calculated by dividing the running distances by 4; cycling distances, by multiplying the running distances by 2.5.

Cooper's 1.5 Mile Test

The time required to run/walk 1.5 miles is also an easy test to use to evaluate your endurance fitness. Standards and fitness categories are given in Table 7–8 for men and Table 7–9 for women.

TABLE 7-8 Standards for Cooper's 1.5 Mile Test (Men)*

CLASSIFI-CATION	AGE GROUPS (YEARS)			
	Under 30	30–39	40–49	50 and up
Very poor	Over 16:01†	Over 16:31†	Over 17:31†	Over 19:01†
Poor	14:01–16:00	14:44–16:30	15:36–17:30	17:01–19:00
Fair	12:01–14:00	12:31–14:45	13:01–15:35	14:31–17:00
Good	10:46–12:00	11:01–12:30	11:31–13:00	12:31–14:30
Excellent	Under 10:45	Under 11:00	Under 11:30	Under 12:30

*From Cooper, K.: *The Aerobics Way,* New York: M. Evans Co., 1977, p. 89.
†Minutes:seconds

TABLE 7–9   Standards for Cooper's 1.5 Mile Test (Women)*

CLASSIFI-CATION	AGE GROUPS (YEARS)			
	Under 30	30–39	40–49	50 and up
Very poor	Over 19:01†	Over 19:31†	Over 20:01†	Over 20:31†
Poor	18:31–19:00	19:01–19:30	19:31–20:00	20:01–20:30
Fair	15:55–18:30	16:31–19:00	17:31–19:30	19:01–20:00
Good	13:31–15:54	14:31–16:30	15:56–17:30	16:31–19:00
Excellent	12:30–13:30	13:00–14:30	13:45–15:55	14:30–16:30

*From Cooper, K.: *The Aerobics Way,* New York: M. Evans Co., 1977, p. 89.
†Minutes:seconds

EVALUATION OF YOUR MUSCULAR FITNESS LEVEL

As with the evaluation of your endurance fitness level, there are several tests available to evaluate your muscular fitness level. Specifically, you will want to evaluate your muscular strength, muscular endurance, and flexibility. Again, whichever test is used should be performed at the beginning of your fitness program and, then again, after 8 to 10 weeks of training.

Muscular Strength Tests

Perhaps the easiest and most convenient way to measure your muscular strength is by the *one-repetition maximum test.* One repetition maximum refers to the maximum amount of weight you can lift just once (only one repetition). The one-repetition maximum load is determined through trial and error. For example, start with a weight that you can lift fairly comfortably, then add weights until you can lift that weight only one time. That will be your one-repetition maximum load. This test can be performed using either the Universal Gym, barbells, or the Nautilus machines. However, whichever apparatus is used to test your strength at the beginning of your strength program should be used for all subsequent tests.

Your strength test should involve a one-repetition maximum test for each group of muscles tested. For example, you will want to select muscle groups from both the upper and lower body. It is suggested that four one-repetition maximum tests be used for the following exercises: (1) the bench press for testing the muscles of the chest and upper arms; (2) press behind the neck for testing the muscles of the shoulders and posterior aspects of the upper arms; (3) the arm curl for the muscles of the anterior aspects of the upper arms; and (4) the leg press for the muscles of the upper legs and hips. Performance of these exercises was described in Chapter 4.

Some guidelines for the optimal strength values for the various muscle groups are presented in Table 7–10. These particular values were obtained using the

TABLE 7–10   Guidelines for the One-Repetition Maximum Strength Test
(in Pounds) for Various Muscle Groups and Body Weights*

BODY WEIGHT (pounds)	BENCH PRESS		PRESS BEHIND NECK		ARM CURL		LEG PRESS	
	Men	Women	Men	Women	Men	Women	Men	Women
80	76	53	55	40	40	30	160	120
100	95	67	70	50	50	35	200	150
120	114	80	80	60	60	40	240	180
140	133	93	95	65	70	50	280	210
160	152	106	110	75	80	60	320	240
180	171	120	120	85	90	65	360	270
200	190	133	135	95	100	70	400	300
220	210	145	150	105	110	75	440	330
240	230	160	160	115	120	85	480	360

*Adapted from Falls, H. B., Baylor, A. M., and Dishman, R. K.: *Essentials of Fitness*. Philadelphia: Saunders College Publishing, 1980, p. 232.

Universal Gym. If Nautilus equipment or barbells are used, the values will undoubtedly be different. Remember, the most important information relative to your own muscular strength program is how much strength you've gained since beginning your program.

Other tests for muscular strength are available but require expensive equipment and, frequently, a technician to operate them. Therefore, they are not generally available so they can be used on a routine basis.

Tests of muscular power

Another muscular capacity that is often improved with strength training is *muscular power*. Muscular power is most often defined as the rate of performing muscular work. Rate, of course, implies time. Therefore, muscular power is performing as much work as possible in the shortest period of time. Sprinting 50 yards is a good example of an activity requiring muscular power. The following are some tests for evaluating your muscular power.

1. Jump and Reach Test. For this test, it is best to use a blackened plywood board, 5 feet long and 1 foot wide, like the one shown in Figure 7–3, that can be mounted on a basketball backstop or a wall. If mounted on the wall, the board should be at least 6 inches out from the wall so that you don't scrape yourself while jumping. To perform the test, first chalk your hands (preferably with magnesium like the gymnasts use). Stand on a line one foot out from the board and reach as high as possible, keeping both heels on the floor. Then jump three times from a crouched position, making a chalk mark on the board at the top of each jump. The distance from the top of the reach mark to the top of the highest jump mark is recorded as your score (to the nearest quarter inch).

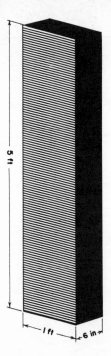

Figure 7–3. Jump and reach board used in the jump and reach test for muscular power.

Your power output can be calculated from your jump reach score and your body weight by using a chart known as the Lewis Nomogram (see Figure 7–4). For example, if your jump-reach score is 24 inches and your body weight is 165 pounds, a ruler is laid across the nomogram touching 24 inches on the distance scale (left) and 165 pounds on the weight scale (right). The power output is read from the center scale — in this case, approximately 952 foot-pounds per second (ft-lb/sec) or about 1.7 horsepower (HP). In other words, your legs have the power of 1.7 horses!

2. The 50-Yard Dash. Perhaps the simplest test to use to evaluate muscular power is the time required to run 50 yards with a 15-yard running start. You'll need a friend with a stopwatch and a marked track to perform this test. Standards for the 50-yard dash for both men and women are shown in Table 7–11.

Muscular Endurance Tests

Muscular endurance tests are not numerous. From a theoretical standpoint, the number of repetitions that can be performed with a certain amount of weight should be the best test for muscular endurance. It has been recommended that, for each muscle group tested, a fixed percentage of 70 percent of the maximum strength be used to evaluate muscular endurance. Your score would be the number of repetitions of that weight you could perform before fatiguing. For

THE LEWIS NOMOGRAM FOR DETERMINING ANAEROBIC POWER FROM
JUMP-REACH SCORE AND BODY WEIGHT

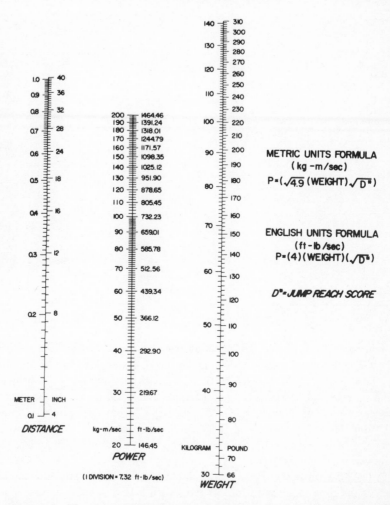

Figure 7–4. The Lewis Nomogram. A person's power output can be determined by knowing the score on the jump reach and the body weight. See text for example. (Courtesy, Office of Naval Research.)

example, suppose on the one-repetition maximum strength test using the bench press that your maximum weight lifted was 150 pounds. To test the muscular endurance of this same muscle group you would count the number of bench press repetitions you could perform using a weight equal to 150 × .7 = 105 pounds. Table 7–12 will help you convert your maximum strength load to a 70-percent load for your endurance test. Although no standards are as yet available,

TABLE 7-11   Guidelines for 50-Yard Dash with 15-Yard Running Start

| CLASSIFI-CATION | MEN Age Groups (years) | | | | |
	15-20	20-30	30-40	40-50	Over 50
Poor	Over 7.1*	Over 7.8*	Over 9.0*	Over 10.8*	Over 13.0*
Fair	7.1-6.8	7.8-7.5	9.0-8.6	10.8-10.3	13.0-12.4
Good	6.7-6.5	7.4-7.1	8.5-8.1	10.2-9.7	12.3-11.6
Excellent	Under 6.5	Under 7.1	Under 8.1	Under 9.7	Under 11.6
CLASSIFI-CATION	WOMEN Age Groups (years)				
	15-20	20-30	30-40	40-50	Over 50
Poor	Over 9.1*	Over 10.0*	Over 11.5*	Over 13.8*	Over 16.5*
Fair	9.1-8.4	10.0-9.2	11.5-10.6	13.8-12.7	16.5-15.2
Good	8.3-7.9	9.1-8.7	10.5-10.0	12.6-12.0	15.1-14.4
Excellent	Under 7.9	Under 8.7	Under 10.0	Under 12.0	Under 14.4

*Seconds

TABLE 7-12   Conversion of Maximum Strength Loads to 70 Percent Loads for Testing of Muscular Endurance

MAXIMUM LOAD (pounds)	70% LOAD (pounds)	MAXIMUM LOAD (pounds)	70% LOAD (pounds)
50	35	280	195
60	42	290	203
70	49	300	210
80	56	310	217
90	63	320	224
100	70	330	231
110	77	340	238
120	84	350	245
130	91	360	252
140	98	370	259
150	105	380	266
160	112	390	273
170	119	400	280
180	126	410	287
190	133	420	294
200	140	430	301
210	147	440	308
220	154	450	315
230	161	460	322
240	168	470	329
250	175	480	336
260	182	490	343
270	189	500	350

if your muscular fitness program is working, you should be able to perform between 10 to 15 repetitions for each muscle group tested using a 70-percent maximum load.

Other popular muscular endurance tests are sit-ups for the abdominal (stomach) muscles and push-ups for the shoulder and upper arm muscles. For sit-ups, lie on the floor with your knees bent. Place your hands behind your neck with fingers clasped and elbows on the floor. Curl to a sitting position (see Figure 4–17, p. 63). The number that you can perform in 2 minutes is your score.

The regular push-up is performed as shown in Figure 7–5. If you are unable to perform a regular push-up, you may try a modification such as doing the push-up from a stool (Figure 7–6), or from the bent-knee position (that is, the knees rather than the toes are on the floor). Again, perform as many push-ups as you can in 2 minutes.

Standards for the number of sit-ups and push-ups that can be performed in 2 minutes are shown in Table 7–13 for men and Table 7–14 for women.

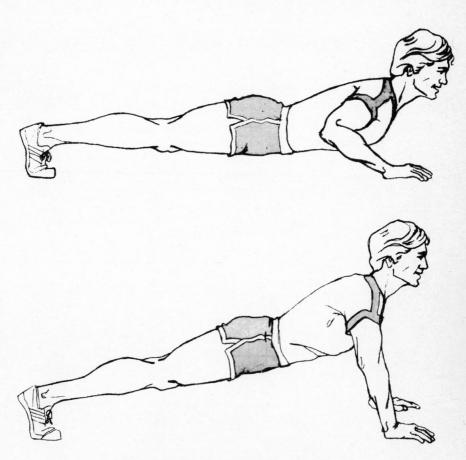

Figure 7–5. Regular push-up from the floor.

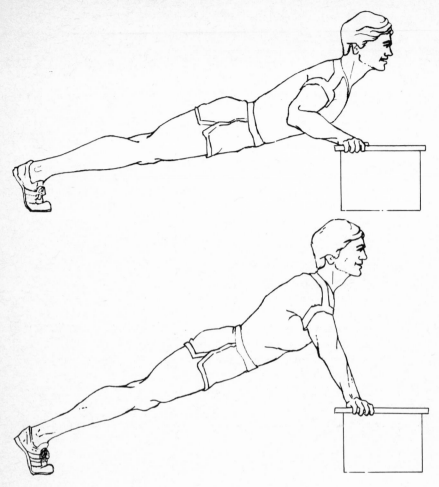

Figure 7–6. Modified push-up from stool.

TABLE 7–13   Guidelines for Number of Sit-ups and Push-ups
by Age Groups (Men)

CLASSIFI-CATION	AGE GROUPS (YEARS)					
	15–25		26–35		Over 35	
	Sit-ups	Push-ups	Sit-ups	Push-ups	Sit-ups	Push-ups
Minimum	10	8	8	7	5	3
Fair	25	15	20	12	15	8
Good	50	25	40	20	30	15
Excellent	80	40	70	30	50	20

TABLE 7–14 Guidelines for Number of Sit-ups and Push-ups
by Age Groups (Women)

| CLASSIFI-CATION | AGE GROUPS (YEARS) | | | | | |
| | 15–25 | | 26–35 | | Over 35 | |
	Sit-ups	Push-ups*	Sit-ups	Push-ups	Sit-ups	Push-ups
Minimum	5	8	4	7	2	3
Fair	15	15	10	12	5	8
Good	20	25	15	20	10	15
Excellent	30	40	20	30	15	20

*Modified push-up such as shown in Fig. 7–6, page 115.

Flexibility tests

Perhaps the simplest test of flexibility of the lower back, hips, and the backs of the upper and lower legs is the ability to touch your toes or the floor from a standing position without bending your knees. A more precise method for such a test is the Wells Sit and Reach Test.

To perform the Wells Sit and Reach Test, sit on the floor with your legs extended forward so that your knees are flat against the floor. Place your feet against a stool or bench to which is attached a scale calibrated in ½-inch units (see Figure 7–7). The scale is attached so that the zero line is at the point where the feet make contact with the stool. The inch lines beyond the zero line are marked +1, +2, +3 and so on, whereas the lines before the zero mark are marked –1, –2, –3 and so forth. With your feet in place, reach forward with your palms down, along the scale. The maximum distance reached is recorded as the measure of your flexibility. Remember, a minus score means that you can't even touch

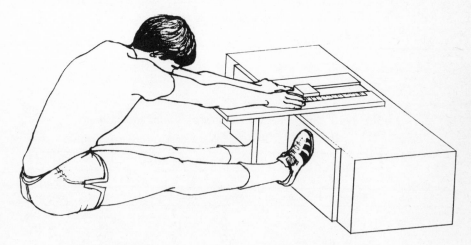

Figure 7-7. The Wells Sit and Reach Test.

your toes, a zero score that you can just barely touch your toes and a positive score signifies that you can reach *beyond* your toes! Obviously, the higher the positive score, the more flexible you are.

Some standards for the Wells Sit and Reach Test are presented in Table 7–15.

EVALUATING YOUR NUTRITIONAL FITNESS AND BODY COMPOSITION

You will recall from Chapters 5 and 6 that nutritional fitness deals with proper selection of foods, good eating habits, and the control of body weight.

Evaluating Your Diet and Eating Habits

It's one thing to know which food groups your foods should be selected from (see p. 73), but it's another to know whether or not you are actually making the proper selection on a day-to-day basis. Therefore, occasionally (e.g., three or four days during one week, once every month), you may want to fill out what is referred to as a "diet diary," in which you write down what you've eaten, how much you've eaten, and how many calories you've taken in per day. An example of one is shown in Table 7–16. Once you've identified the kind of food, compare it to the four food group list given in Table 5–3 on page 74.

The diet diary can also be used to evaluate your eating habits. For instance, in our example (Table 7–16) notice how the caloric intake is fairly evenly spread throughout the day. Also notice that the snacks consist of nutritious foods rather than the more popular but less nutritious junk foods. The total number of calories taken in during the day may also be monitored with the diet diary. Remember, the caloric values for various foods are contained in Tables 6–4 and 6–5, pages 86 and 93.

TABLE 7–15   Standards for the Wells Sit and Reach Test for Flexibility

FLEXIBILITY RATING	SIT AND REACH SCORE (inches)
Poor	−3 or more
Fair	−1 to −2
Average	0 to +3
Good	+4 to +6
Excellent	+7 or greater

**TABLE 7–16   The Diet Diary for Evaluating Selection of Foods,
Caloric Intake, and Eating Habits**

Breakfast   Calories
3/4 cup (6 oz.) orange juice   85
2 soft boiled eggs   160
3 slices whole wheat toast   130
2 tsp. margarine   35
1 glass (8 oz.) skim milk   90
                                                            Total   500

Lunch
1 ham + cheese on white bread   350
1 tsp. pickle relish   20
1/2 sliced tomato   13
10 potato chips   115
1 medium apple   80
1 glass (8 oz.) skim milk   90
                                                            Total   668

Dinner
1 serving (3½ oz.) roasted chicken   170
3/4 cup (6 oz.) white rice   170
6 brussels sprouts   45
lettuce salad (½ head)   30
1½ tsp. french dressing   100
1 slice gingerbread   170
1 glass (8 oz.) skim milk   90
                                                            Total   775

Snacks
1 banana (10:30 AM)   100
1 carton fruit flavored yogurt (8 PM)   225
3/4 cup (6 oz.) grape juice (9:30 PM)   120

                                                            Total   445

                                                    Daily total   2388

Appraising Your Body Composition

Body composition, as mentioned in an earlier chapter, refers to the component parts of the body. For our purposes, there are two components to consider: (1) body fat; and (2) fat-free weight or lean body weight.

You can't evaluate your body composition with just a bathroom scale. More sophisticated methods are required. The most sophisticated method involves underwater weighing. While this method is most accurate, it is least accessible to most of us. The procedure requires a special tank and scale so that your body weight can be recorded while you are totally submerged under water (see Figure 7–8). It also requires special equipment to measure the volume of air in your lungs while you are submerged.

An alternative but less accurate way to assess your body composition is by measuring the thickness of your skinfolds at specific sites on the body. This is the so-called "pinch an inch" test. As shown in Figure 7–9, the skinfold measurements are taken with an instrument called a *skinfold caliper*. The caliper shown in the figure is expensive, around $200. However, you can obtain a good, reliable skinfold caliper, free of charge, from Ross Laboratories, 625 Cleveland Ave., Columbus, Ohio 43216.

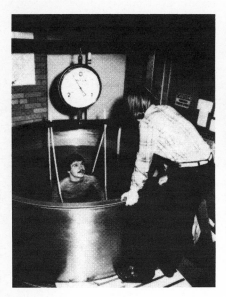 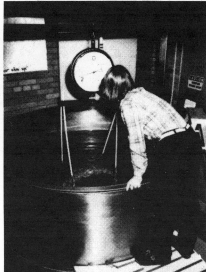

Figure 7–8. Underwater weighing tank for determining percentage of body fat. (Photographs by Tom Malloy, Courtesy, Department of Photography, The Ohio State University.)

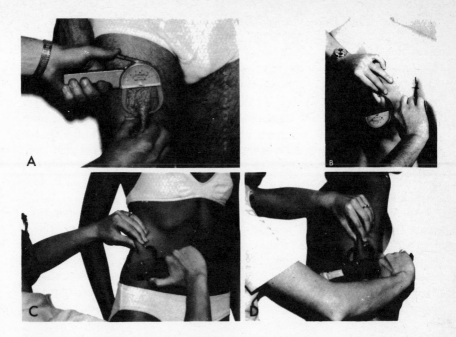

Figure 7-9. Skinfold measurements. A, Thigh (men); B, Subscapular (men); C, Suprailiac (women); D, Triceps (women). These skinfolds should be used with Figure 7-10 (men) and Figure 7-11 (women) for determination of percent body fat.

As the name implies, skinfolds measure folds of skin only — no muscle tissue should be included. Since a large portion of body fat is stored under the skin, the thickness of the skinfold reflects your body fat content.

For men, two skinfolds, the subscapular (back of shoulder) and the thigh (front of upper leg) can be used to estimate body fat. For women, two different skinfolds are used: the suprailiac (above the hip), and triceps (back of the upper arm). These skinfold sites are shown in Figure 7-9. The skinfolds are measured in millimeters* on the right side of the body and you'll need someone to measure you. (In other words, you can't measure yourself.) As shown in Figure 7-9, hold the skinfold firmly between your thumb and index finger. Then, place the caliper on the skinfold as closely as possible to your thumb and finger (usually about ½ inch). The exact locations of the four skinfolds mentioned above are:

For men

1. Thigh Skinfold (Figure 7-9A). Stand relaxed. Pick up the skinfold in the vertical (up and down) plane on the front surface of the thigh, midway between the hip and knee joint.

---

*One inch equals 25.4 millimeters.

2. Subscapular Skinfold (Figure 7–9B).   Stand relaxed. Pick up the skinfold just below the point of the shoulder blade (scapula), in a slight slant running laterally in the natural fold of the skin.

For women

1. Suprailiac Skinfold (Figure 7–9C).   Stand relaxed. Pick up the skinfold just above the top of the hip bone (ilium) at the middle of the side of the body.

2. Triceps Skinfold (Figure 7–9D).   Stand with right elbow flexed 90 degrees. Locate the level on the back of the upper arm halfway between the shoulder and the tip of the elbow and then relax the arm at the side. At the level previously located, pick up the skinfold in the vertical (up and down) plane.

Once the skinfolds have been measured, they may be applied to the graphs found in Figure 7–10 for men or Figure 7–11 for women to determine your percentage of body fat. Here is an example of how to use the graphs: Suppose you are a man and your thigh skinfold is 16 millimeters and your subscapular skinfold is 12 millimeters. Lay a ruler across the graph in Figure 7–10, touching 16 millimeters on the left scale and 12 millimeters on the right scale. The percentage of body fat is then read from the center scale — in this case, it is 14 percent body fat.

Some standards for the percentage of body fat for college-age men and women are presented in Table 7–17.

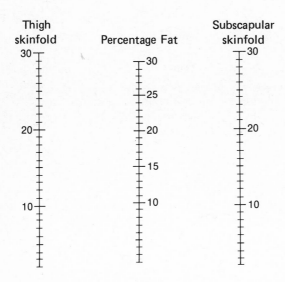

Figure 7–10.   Graph for determining percent body fat from thigh skinfold (left scale) and subscapular skinfold (right scale) in young men. To use, connect skinfold readings with straight edge, then read percent body fat from center scale. (Adapted from Sloan, A. W., and Weir, J. B. de V.: Nomograms for the prediction of body density and body fat from skinfold measurements. *J. Appl. Physiol.* **28**:221–222, 1970.)

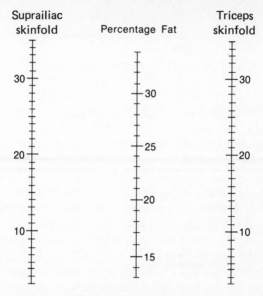

Figure 7-11. Graph for determining percent body fat from suprailiac skinfold (left scale) and triceps skinfold (right scale) in young women. To use, connect skinfold readings with straight edge, then read percent body fat from center scale. (Adapted from Sloan, A. W., and Weir, J. B. de V.: Nomograms for the prediction of body density and body fat from skinfold measurements. *J. Appl. Physiol.* 28:221–222, 1970.)

What's Your Ideal Body Weight?

The standards given in Table 7-17 are based on measurements taken at random from a group of college students. The average value, therefore, does not necessarily represent an ideal body composition. On the contrary, the ideal percentage of body fat for both sexes would be below average, that is, for men, 12 percent, and for women, 18 percent. Once you know what your percentage of body fat actually is, you can calculate your ideal body weight as follows:

1. *Determine your fat weight.* This is done by multiplying your total body weight times your fraction of body fat.

TABLE 7-17 Body Fat Standards*

CLASSIFICATION	MALE (%)	FEMALE (%)
Very low fat	7 – 9.9	14 – 16.9
Low fat	10 – 12.9	17 – 19.9
Average fat	13 – 16.9	20 – 23.9
Above average fat	17 – 19.9	24 – 26.9
Very high fat	20 – 24.9	27 – 29.9
Obese	25 and higher	30 and higher

*Based on data from Sloan, A. W.: "Estimation of body fat in young men." *J. Appl. Physiol.* 23:311–315, 1967, and Sloan, A. W., Burt, J. J., and Blyth, C. S.: "Estimation of body fat in young women." *J. Appl. Physiol.* 17:967–970, 1962.

Example (Women)

> Total body weight = 145 pounds
> % body fat = 28%
> fat weight = 28% of 145 = **40.6 pounds**

2. *Determine your fat-free or lean body weight.* This is done by subtracting your fat weight from your total body weight.

Example

> Lean body weight = 145 – 40.6 = **104.4 pounds**

3. *Add to your lean body weight an amount of fat that represents the ideal body fat percentage.* As mentioned earlier, for women, this is 18 percent and for men, 12 percent. The way this is done is by dividing the lean body weight by 0.82 (100% – 18% or 1 – .18) for women, and 0.88 (100% – 12% or 1 – .12) for men.

Example

> Ideal weight = 104.4/.82 = **127.3 pounds.**

This means that you need to lose 145 – 127.3 = 17.7 or 18 pounds. You should, of course follow the guidelines outlined in Chapter 6 for losing body fat (p. 97).

To help you in calculating your ideal body weight when you know your lean body weight, see Table 7–18.

TABLE 7–18   Ideal Body Weights for Men and Women
from Lean Body Weights

Lean Body Weight (pounds)	MEN Ideal Body Weight (pounds)*	WOMEN Ideal Body Weight (pounds)†
70		85.3
80		97.6
90	102.3	109.7
100	113.6	122.0
110	125.0	134.1
120	136.4	146.3
130	147.7	158.5
140	159.1	170.7
150	170.4	182.9
160	181.8	195.1
170	193.2	
180	204.5	
190	215.9	
200	227.3	

*Based on 12% body fat.
†Based on 18% body fat.

A FINAL NOTE ABOUT YOUR
APPRAISAL PROGRAM

Many tables of standards for various tests have been presented. However, please don't regard these standards as levels you must achieve. Everyone is different — very few people are statistically average — so there will always be a range of satisfactory performance. What is most important is your own progress. Use the tests to measure your progress as you train, and use the tables only as guidelines. As you become more fit, you will be able to set your own standards for your own personal fitness. If you have to temporarily stop exercising for some reason, those standards will give you something to aim for as you renew your efforts. You make the determination about yourself — you are your own best guide to personal fitness and health.

8 □ Answers to Commonly Asked Questions About Fitness

The main purpose of this chapter is to present to you answers to frequently asked questions about exercise and fitness. Sometimes, although it's never intentional, some very important questions never get answered during the course of writing a textbook. This chapter is written, therefore, to answer some of your questions about fitness that may not have been answered already.

The questions are arranged according to subject area as best as possible. Generally the subject areas follow the outline of the book. Since many questions and answers include different subject areas, there is some overlapping. Therefore, if you can't find a particular question and answer under one subject heading, look for it under a related heading.

Exercise, Fitness, and Health

Question: What is the leading killer among diseases in the United States?

Answer: Of all deaths in the United States, more than half are due to cardiovascular diseases.

Question: What are cardiovascular diseases and what causes them?

Answer: Cardiovascular diseases affect the heart and blood vessels of the circulatory system. The most common cardiovascular diseases are heart attack or coronary heart disease, which is the number one killer, stroke, and hypertension (high blood pressure). The major cause of cardiovascular disease is atherosclerosis, a slow, progressive disease that causes narrowing of the arteries in the heart as well as those throughout the rest of the body.

Question: What is a heart attack?

Answer: A heart attack occurs when the blood flow through an artery supplying blood to the heart muscle is blocked (usually as a result of
atherosclerosis). When this occurs, that part of the heart muscle
dies that was supplied with blood by that artery.

Question: What are some of the risk factors associated with heart attack or
coronary heart disease?

Answer: There are nine currently known risk factors: (1) age — the older
you are, the greater your risk of a heart attack; (2) heredity —
people who suffer heart attack generally have a family history of
heart attack; (3) obesity; (4) cigarette smoking; (5) lack of exercise;
(6) high blood cholesterol levels; (7) high blood pressure (hypertension); (8) sex — the risk of coronary heart disease is greater in
men; and (9) stress.

Question: Which risk factors are most important?

Answer: The three most important risk factors are (1) cigarette smoking;
(2) high blood pressure; and (3) high blood levels of cholesterol.

Question: How does regular exercise protect against coronary heart disease?

Answer: Regular exercise can lead to decreases in blood pressure, blood
cholesterol levels, obesity, and temporary relief from stress. You'll
notice that all of these are risk factors of coronary heart disease.
Therefore, simply by exercising on a regular basis, five of the nine
risk factors can be lowered!

Question: What is fitness?

Answer: Fitness implies a physiological or functional capacity that allows
for an improved quality of life. It has five components: (1) cardiorespiratory or endurance fitness; (2) muscular fitness; (3) nutritional
fitness; (4) mental and emotional fitness; and (5) motor fitness.

The Physiology of Fitness

Question: Of all the physiological systems in the body, which ones are most
important to the understanding of fitness?

Answer: Three physiological systems seem to be most directly related to
fitness: (1) metabolism, or the energy-producing system; (2) the
heart-lung or cardiovascular and respiratory systems; and (3) the
muscular system.

Question: What is metabolism and how does it relate to fitness?

Answer: Metabolism refers to the various series of chemical reactions involved in energy production that take place within the body. By
understanding how energy is produced, exercise programs can be
developed so as to yield specific kinds of fitness capacities (e.g.,
heart-lung or endurance fitness).

Question: What does aerobic metabolism mean?

Answer: This refers to the series of chemical reactions involved in energy
production that requires oxygen in order to be completed (aerobic

= with oxygen). Aerobic metabolism supplies most of the energy needed during exercises continued for relatively long periods of time, such as running a marathon. It is involved in endurance fitness.

Question: What does anaerobic metabolism mean?

Answer: Anaerobic metabolism refers to the series of chemical reactions involved in energy production that does not require oxygen in order to be completed (anaerobic = without oxygen). Anaerobic metabolism supplies most of the energy needed during high-intensity but short-duration exercises, such as sprinting.

Question: What is ATP and how is it related to metabolism?

Answer: ATP is an abbreviation for a chemical compound found in the body called adenosine triphosphate. When it's broken down, a lot of energy is released. This energy is the only energy that can be directly used for the body's various functions, including muscular contraction. Other forms of chemical energy, such as those made available through aerobic and anaerobic metabolism, must be transferred into the ATP form before they can be utilized by the muscle cells.

Question: What is the relationship between energy production and nutritional fitness?

Answer: The link between the metabolic system and nutrition is easy to see. For example, the foodstuffs, carbohydrates, fats, and proteins, when chemically broken down, provide the energy that is transferred into the ATP form. Also, when oxygen is taken in to help break down the foodstuffs, calories are expended, hence the relationship to body weight.

Question: How are the circulatory and respiratory systems related to fitness?

Answer: The major job of the circulatory and respiratory systems is to deliver oxygen to the muscles. This is important in that it provides the ability to perform exercises of long duration. In other words, the circulatory and respiratory systems provide the physiological basis for one of the components of fitness, heart-lung or endurance fitness.

Question: What do cardiac output, stroke volume, and heart rate mean?

Answer: Cardiac output refers to the amount of blood put out by the heart (cardiac = heart) in one minute. Stroke volume of the heart refers to how much blood is put out by the heart with each beat. The heart rate refers to the number of times the heart beats in one minute. Multiplying the stroke volume times the heart rate equals the cardiac output. All of these factors increase during exercise.

Question: How many kinds of muscle are there in the human body?

Answer: There are three kinds of muscle in the body: (1) heart muscle; (2) smooth muscles, which are found in the walls of the blood vessels, in the gastrointestinal tract, and in other internal organs; and (3) skeletal muscles, which move the bony skeleton to produce movement.

Question: What are fast- and slow-twitch muscle fibers?

Answer: Fast-twitch muscle fibers have a high capacity for anaerobic metabolism and a low capacity for aerobic metabolism. Slow-twitch fibers have a high capacity for aerobic metabolism and a low capacity for anaerobic metabolism. As a result, slow-twitch fibers are mainly used for endurance activities, whereas fast-twitch fibers are mostly used for sprintlike activities.

Question: How many types of muscular contraction are there and how do they differ?

Answer: There are four basic types of muscular contractions: (1) an isotonic contraction, in which the muscle shortens as it develops force or tension; (2) an isometric contraction, in which the muscle develops force but does not change its length; (3) an eccentric contraction, in which the muscle lengthens as it develops force; and (4) an isokinetic contraction, in which the muscle shortens and develops tension such as in an isotonic contraction but at a constant speed.

Endurance Fitness Programs

Question: What is endurance fitness?

Answer: Cardiorespiratory or endurance fitness is defined as the capacity or ability of the heart-lung system to deliver blood and thus oxygen to the working muscles during prolonged physical activity or exercise.

Question: What physiological and other changes result from endurance fitness programs?

Answer: Several changes occur as a result of endurance fitness programs. All of the changes help promote health and reduce the risk of coronary heart disease. Here they are: (1) improvement in the transport of oxygen by the heart and lungs to the muscles; (2) increased ability of muscles to use oxygen; (3) increased circulatory efficiency; (4) increased blood vessel size and capillarization of the heart muscle; (5) reduced possibility of blood clot; (6) reduced occurrence of cardiac dysrhythmias; (7) improved tolerance to stress; and (8) reduction in other coronary heart disease risk factors such as decreases in obesity, blood pressure, and blood cholesterol levels.

Question: What is meant by an "exercise prescription"?

Answer: Your physician prescribes medicine that is given to reduce or minimize symptoms caused by disease. An exercise prescription is similar. In this case, the "disease" is a low endurance fitness level, and some of the "symptoms" are breathlessness upon exertion, chronic fatigue, and overweight. The correct prescription, of course, is regular participation in an exercise program involving activities that are carried out over prolonged periods of time (15 to 60 minutes per day) and that sufficiently stress the heart-lung system. An exercise prescription starts with a good medical examination and then sets the limits for the frequency, intensity, and duration of your exercise program.

Question: How many times a week should you exercise?

Answer: Exercise must be performed on a regular basis in order to assure improvement in your endurance fitness. Therefore, you should exercise three to five days per week, for example, on Monday, Wednesday, and Friday, or Tuesday, Thursday, and Saturday, or Monday through Friday.

Question: How hard should you exercise?

Answer: The intensity of your exercise should be judged by how high your heart rate is during the exercise session. During your exercise session, your heart rate, or target heart rate as it's usually called, should be between 60 percent and 90 percent of your maximum heart rate reserve. The heart rate reserve is the percent difference between your resting and maximum heart rates added to your resting heart rate.

Question: How can you determine your heart rate?

Answer: Your resting heart rate is fairly easy to determine. You can count your pulse at any of several arteries, for example, at the wrist, the neck, or the temple.

Your maximum heart rate, however, is not easy to directly obtain. This requires a graded exercise stress test performed on either a treadmill or bicycle ergometer. Without a stress test, your maximum heart rate can be estimated by subtracting your age from 220 (maximum heart rate = 220 − age).

It is not possible to accurately take your pulse during exercise. However, a pulse count obtained in a 6- or 10-second span immediately following exercise is a reasonable indicator of what the heart rate was during exercise. Remember, a 6-second pulse count would be multiplied by 10, a 10-second count by 6, and a 15-second count by 4 to convert to beats per minute.

Question: How long should you exercise?

Answer: During your workout, the exercise should be performed continuously at the proper intensity for 15 to 60 minutes. Duration is dependent upon the intensity of the exercise, thus, lower intensity exercises should be conducted over a longer period of time. A lower to moderate intensity exercise of longer duration, as opposed to a higher intensity exercise of shorter duration, is recommended for the nonathletic adult. Remember, the duration of your workout should be based on time, that is, 15 to 60 minutes, not on the completion of a certain distance (miles).

Question: What kind of exercise should you perform?

Answer: The type of exercise you perform during your training program should involve the large muscle groups, be maintained continuously, and be rhythmical and aerobic in nature. Good examples of these kinds of exercises are walking, running and jogging, bicycling, and swimming.

Question: What kinds of exercises should you do during your warm-up before and warm- (cool) down after your workout?

Answer: Three types of warm-up and/or warm-down activities are recommended: (1) stretching exercises for flexibility and for possible protection against muscular injury and soreness; (2) calisthenics for development of muscular strength and endurance; and (3) brief formal activity of the type used in your endurance program. Stretching should be considered most important for the warm-up, whereas brief formal activity and stretching, in that order, are best for the warm-down.

Question: What precautions, if any, should you take when working out outdoors on a hot day?

Answer: Exercise coupled with hot weather can lead to loss of body water (dehydration) due to profuse sweating and to heat illness due to overheating. Both conditions can lead to serious health problems, even death. Here are some guidelines on how to avoid heat illness: (1) drink plenty of water by drinking small amounts (3 to 6 ounces) frequently; (2) do not take salt tablets, but be sure to salt your food during meals; (3) wear appropriate clothing — sweatsuits of any kind should *not* be worn under any circumstances when exercising in hot weather; (4) work out during the coolest parts of the day (morning or evening); and (5) on extremely hot days, don't be afraid to cut back or skip your workout altogether.

Muscular Fitness Programs

Question: What is muscular fitness?

Answer: Muscular fitness has three subcomponents: (1) muscular strength, which is the force a muscle or muscle group can exert during contraction; (2) muscular endurance, which is the length of time a muscle or muscle group can continue to exert force without fatiguing; and (3) joint flexibility, which is the range of motion possible about a joint over which a muscle spans.

Question: What physiological and other changes result from muscular fitness programs?

Answer: The changes include (1) increased muscular strength; (2) increased muscular endurance; (3) increased muscular size; (4) increased flexibility; (5) decreased total and relative body fat; (6) increased total body muscle mass; and (7) improved performance of some skills.

Question: Do muscular fitness programs develop endurance fitness?

Answer: No, only muscular fitness. Endurance fitness is developed as discussed earlier (p. 128).

Question: What kind of exercise program can best develop muscular fitness?

Answer: The best program for developing muscular strength, muscular endurance, and flexibility is a weight training, weight lifting, or weight resistance program. Such programs consist of muscular contractions performed against resistance as when lifting free weights (barbells) or weight stacks that are attached to specific weight lifting equipment such as Nautilus and Universal Gym.

Question: How much weight should you lift?

Answer: In the first two weeks of your weight training program, pick a weight that you can lift 15 times before fatiguing. When you are able to do 20 repetitions, increase the weight 5 pounds or one plate if you are using a machine with a weight stack. After two weeks, use a weight which you can properly lift 8 to 10 times, and do not increase the weight until you can lift it 12 to 15 times.

Question: How do you select a weight that you can lift a certain number of times?

Answer: The simplest way is by "trial and error." Start with light or moderate weight, then add weight as necessary. Rest between trials.

Question: How many days per week should you lift?

Answer: You should lift three days per week with a rest day between each workout. For example, lift on Monday, Wednesday, and Friday and rest on the other days of the week.

Question: Which muscle groups should you exercise?

Answer: You should exercise all the major muscle groups as follows: (1) upper legs and hips; (2) chest and upper arms; (3) back and posterior (back) aspects of legs; (4) lower legs and ankles; (5) shoulders and posterior aspects of the upper arms; (6) stomach; and (7) anterior (front) aspects of upper arms.

Question: In what order should the muscle groups be exercised?

Answer: In the order given in the last answer, that is, the large muscle groups first, then the smaller groups.

Question: Which equipment should you use — barbells, Nautilus, or Universal Gym?

Answer: It really doesn't matter. You can even mix them so that some exercises are done with barbells, some with Nautilus, and some with Universal.

Question: Is a weight training program the only way to improve flexibility?

Answer: No. Although flexibility can be increased through weight training programs, stretching exercises can also improve your flexibility.

Nutritional Fitness

Question: What is nutritional fitness?

Answer: Nutritional fitness is concerned with the proper selection of foods with regard to their nutrient and caloric values as well as with proper eating habits.

Question: What are food nutrients?

Answer: There are three classes of food nutrients: (1) energy nutrients; (2) vitamins and minerals; and (3) water.

Question: What are energy nutrients?

Answer: The energy nutrients are proteins, fats, and carbohydrates. When they are metabolically (chemically) broken down, energy is released, some of which is captured as ATP.

Question: What are vitamins and minerals?

Answer: Vitamins serve as essential parts of enzymes or coenzymes that are vital to the metabolism of the energy nutrients. The water-soluble vitamins are Vitamin C and the B-complex vitamins, whereas the fat-soluble vitamins are A, D, E, and K. Minerals are compounds found in trace amounts in the body and are also important to proper bodily function. Calcium, phosphorous, potassium, sodium, iron, and iodine are a few of the more important required minerals.

Question: How important is water?

Answer: Water is the most essential food nutrient for human life. It is important in the regulation of body temperature and is the medium in which all the body processes occur.

Question: What are your food requirements?

Answer: Food requirements are based on your nutritional and caloric needs. Nutritional needs can be met if a certain proportion of the total calories taken in are derived from each of the three foodstuffs as follow: protein, 10 to 15 percent; fat, 25 to 30 percent; and carbohydrates, 55 to 60 percent. Your caloric needs should be approximately equal to the calories you expend for body maintenance and physical activities. When more calories are taken in than expended, body weight increases, and when less calories are taken in than expended, body weight decreases.

Question: What are saturated and unsaturated fats and how do they relate to coronary heart disease?

Answer: Saturated fats are in a solid form at room temperature and include animal fats such as those found in meats. Eggs and dairy products also contain high levels of saturated fats. Eating large amounts of saturated fats is not recommended since it is thought to lead to high blood cholesterol levels, atherosclerosis, and cardiovascular disease. Unsaturated fats, which are not associated with cardiovascular disease, are in a liquid form at room temperature. They are found in vegetable oils such as peanut oil, corn oil, and soybean oil.

Question: During exercise training, should you increase your dietary intake of protein?

Answer: No. In adults, the protein requirement during heavy exercise is not significantly increased. Therefore, the consumption of excessive quantities of protein, particularly in the forms of pills and powders, during heavy exercise is neither required nor recommended.

Question: Are vitamin and mineral supplements necessary during periods of increased physical activity?

Answer: No. The one exception might be the requirement for iron, which is found in red blood cells and is responsible for the oxygen-carrying ability of the blood. This is particularly true for women. A note of caution: anyone contemplating taking iron supplements should first consult a physician.

Question: Are there any special foods you should eat before exercising or competing?

Answer: No, there are no foods that, when taken several hours prior to physical activity, will lead to "super" performances. There are, however, certain foods that should probably be avoided on the day of intense exercise or competition. Examples of these are fats and meats, gas-forming foods, "greasy" foods, and highly seasoned foods. Probably the best food to eat before exercising is carbohydrate.

Diet, Exercise, and Body Weight Control

Question: What is meant by body composition?

Answer: Body composition refers to two major component parts of the body: (1) body fat, and (2) fat-free weight or lean body weight. Lean body weight reflects mainly muscle weight or mass. The average body fat for college-age men is 15 percent; whereas the average for college-age women is 26 percent.

Question: Is the percentage of body fat in women linked to menstrual irregularities?

Answer: Yes, there are some who believe that body fat values below 15 percent in women might be associated with the cessation of menstruation or secondary amenorrhea. However, it must be pointed out that menstruation is not significantly affected, whatever the percentage of body fat, by exercise and training. Also, menstruation does not always adversely affect physical performance.

Question: What is obesity or overfatness?

Answer: Obesity or overfatness refers to the above-average amount of fat contained in the body. Generally, anyone whose total body weight is in excess of 25 percent of his or her college age weight is considered to be obese or overfat.

Question: What do you have to do in order to lose body fat?

Answer: First, more calories need to be expended than are taken in through the diet. It requires an excess expenditure of 3500 kilocalories in order to lose one pound of pure fat. In order to maximize your caloric deficit and insure fat loss rather than lean body (muscle) loss, your weight loss program should combine dieting and exercising. For health reasons, you should not lose more than four pounds per week.

Question: Are the claims of many health spas that you can lose a lot of "inches" and a lot of weight in just a few days true?

Answer: Some of them are probably true. However, it must be understood
              that the "inches" represent a sum of inches lost from several body
              areas. These losses, as well as any loss of total body weight, are a
              result of fluid shifts and the loss of body water, not fat. Of course,
              this kind of weight loss is neither permanent nor does it significantly
              affect your body composition. In fact, if continued for long periods
              of time, it can even be dangerous. Since the loss of body fat is a
              relatively slow process, beware of any claims for rapid weight loss!

Question: What is spot reducing and how does it work?

Answer: It doesn't! Many people believe that by exercising a specific body
              area or spot, the fat stored there will be selectively reduced. That is
              not true. Regardless of which body area is exercised, the fat stores
              are reduced all over the body, not just selectively from one area.
              Spot reducing is a myth!

Question: What do you have to do in order to gain muscle mass or lean body
              weight?

Answer: In order to gain one pound of muscle mass, an excess dietary intake
              of 2500 kilocalories is required. An excess of this size should *not*
              be taken in one day, rather, excess intake should be no greater than
              1000 to 1500 kilocalories. To ensure that the excess calories will
              be laid down primarily as muscle and not fat, a weight resistance
              program should be performed three days per week.

Appraising Your Fitness Programs

Question: What is the purpose of appraising your fitness programs?

Answer: Evaluation of your progress will help you in maintaining both
              interest and motivation in your fitness programs. Good evaluation
              will also help you to adjust your fitness programs so the most bene-
              ficial results can be obtained.

Question: Should you have a medical examination before you begin a fitness
              program?

Answer: Absolutely. No one should begin an exercise program without first
              obtaining his or her physician's approval. In addition to the physical
              examination, your physician may wish to conduct an exercise
              "stress test." Such a test involves recording your heart rate and
              blood pressure and taking an electrocardiogram (tracing of the elec-
              trical acitivity of the heart muscle). The physician may also check
              how much oxygen you consume while seated and standing during
              and following exercise.

Question: How can you evaluate your endurance fitness?

Answer: The best way is by direct measurement of your maximal oxygen
              consumption; however, it is the least accessible method for you.
              The most practical ways to evaluate your endurance fitness are
              measurement of either your resting, exercise, or recovery heart
              rates. An increase in endurance fitness usually causes your resting

heart rate and your heart rate during and following a given amount of exercise to be lower than they were before you started your fitness program. Therefore, periodic comparison of your heart rate over the course of your endurance fitness program is a good way to evaluate your progress.

Other ways to evaluate your endurance fitness involve how fast you can run 1½ miles or how many miles you can travel in 12 minutes.

Question: How can you evaluate your muscular fitness?

Answer: You will want to evaluate your muscular strength, muscular endurance, and flexibility. The easiest way to measure strength is to see how much weight you can lift just once. You'll need to do this for each muscle group tested.

Muscular endurance can be evaluated by how many repetitions a muscle group can perform while lifting a load that is 70 percent of the maximum load that can be lifted by that muscle group just once. Again, you will need to do this for each muscle group you wish to test. Other popular muscular endurance tests are bent-knee sit-ups for the stomach muscles and push-ups for the shoulder and upper arm muscles. The number of each that you can perform in two minutes is your score.

Flexibility of the lower back, hips, and the backs of the upper and lower legs can be evaluated by whether or not you can touch your toes while keeping your legs straight. This is referred to as the Wells Sit and Reach Test.

Question: How can you evaluate your diet and eating habits?

Answer: You'll need to keep a diet diary for three or four days from one week, once a month. In your diet diary you write down what you've eaten, how much you've eaten, and how many calories you've taken in each day. In this way, you can compare the kind of foods you select to the basic four food groups, how many times you eat each day, and how many calories you are eating.

Question: How can you assess your body composition?

Answer: Probably the most accurate way is by underwater weighing. However, this is also the least practical method. An alternative but less accurate way to assess your body composition is by measuring the thickness of your skinfolds at specific sites on the body.

Question: What is a skinfold and how is it measured?

Answer: A skinfold measures the thickness of your skin and of any fat that is stored under the skin. In this way skinfold thickness reflects your body fat content. Skinfolds are measured with special instruments called skinfold calipers. Knowing the skinfold thickness from several areas of the body, your percentage of body fat can be estimated with the help of specially constructed graphs called nomograms.

Question: What is your ideal body weight?
Answer: Your ideal body weight is based on your lean body weight, which
              is your total body weight minus your fat weight. For men, the
              ideal body weight is the lean body weight plus 12 percent fat,
              whereas for women it's the lean body weight plus 18 percent fat.
              These values can be calculated by dividing your lean body weight
              by 0.88 if you are a man and by 0.82 if you are a woman.

Glossary

A-band — The dark striations of the myofibril.

Adenosine triphosphate (ATP) — A complex chemical compound formed with the energy released from food and stored in all cells, particularly muscle cells. Only with energy released from the breakdown of this compound can the cell perform its function.

Actin — A protein contained in muscle and involved in muscular contraction.

Adipocyte — A fat cell; a cell that stores fat.

Adipose tissue — Fat tissue.

Aerobic — In the presence of oxygen.

Alveolar-capillary membrane — The site in the lung where gas exchange between air and blood occurs.

Alveoli — Tiny terminal air sacs in the lungs.

Amino acids — Nitrogen-containing compounds that form the building blocks of proteins.

Anaerobic — In the absence of oxygen.

Aneurysm — Blood-filled pouch that balloons out from a weak spot in an artery wall.

Arterial blood — Blood high in oxygen and low in carbon dioxide.

Atherosclerosis — A slow, progressive disease involving the narrowing of blood vessels, usually arteries.

Blood pressure — The driving force that moves blood through the circulatory system. Systolic pressure (the higher pressure) is obtained when blood is ejected into the arteries; diastolic pressure (the lower pressure) is obtained when the blood drains from the arteries.

Body composition — The component parts of the body, mainly fat and fat-free weight or lean body weight.

Caloric deficit — Expending more calories through activity than are taken in through the diet.

Calorie — A unit of work or energy equal to the amount of heat required to raise the temperature of one gram of water 1 degree centigrade.

Carbohydrate — A chemical compound containing carbon, hydrogen, and oxygen; one of the basic foodstuffs.

Cardiac output — The amount of blood pumped in one minute by the heart; the product of the heart rate and stroke volume.

Cardiorespiratory — Pertaining to the circulatory and respiratory systems.

Cardiorespiratory fitness — The ability of the heart-lung system to deliver blood and oxygen to the working muscles during prolonged physical exercise.

Cardiovascular disease — Afflictions of the heart and blood vessels.

Central nervous system — The brain and spinal cord.

137

Cholesterol — A fatlike substance found in animal fats and linked to athero-sclerosis as a possible cause.

Coronary heart disease — Afflictions of the heart and its blood vessels; a cardio-vascular disease.

Cross bridges — Tiny projections extending from the myosin filaments in the myofibrils of skeletal muscle.

Dehydration — The condition resulting from excessive loss of body water.

Eccentric contraction — Muscular contraction in which the muscle lengthens while developing tension or force.

Electrocardiogram — A recording of the electrical activity of the heart.

Emotional fitness — Ability to cope with tension and stresses encountered on a daily basis.

Endomysium — The connective tissue that surrounds a muscle fiber or cell.

Endurance fitness — Same as cardiorespiratory fitness.

Energy — The capacity or ability to perform work.

Energy nutrients — Foods that when broken down release energy, some of which is captured as ATP; protein, fats, and carbohydrates.

Epimysium — A connective tissue that surrounds the entire muscle.

Exercise prescription — The quantity and quality of exercise to be performed in a fitness program.

Fast-twitch fiber — A muscle fiber characterized by fast contraction time, high anaerobic metabolism, and low aerobic metabolism.

Fat — A foodstuff containing glycerol and fatty acids; in the body, the soft tis-sue stored in fat cells.

Fat cell — An adipocyte.

Fat-free weight — That portion of the body weight remaining when the weight of body fat is subtracted from the total body weight; mainly the weight of the skeletal muscles.

Fitness — A physiological or functional capacity that allows for an improved quality of life.

Flexibility — The range of motion about a joint over which a muscle spans.

Food nutrients — Energy nutrients, vitamins and minerals, and water.

Foodstuff — A substance suitable for food; carbohydrate, protein, and fat.

Glucose — Sugar; a carbohydrate.

Glycogen — The storage form of glucose in the human body.

Heat illness — Incapacitation from excessively high body temperature.

Heart attack — Death of a part of the heart muscle caused by a lack of blood flow; coronary heart disease.

Heart rate — The number of times the heart beats per minute.

Hypertension — High blood pressure.

Hypertrophy — An increase in the size of a cell such as a muscle cell.

Hyperthermia — Excessively high body temperature.

I-band — The light striations of the myofibril.

Isokinetic contraction — A maximal isotonic contraction performed at constant speed over the full range of joint motion.

Isometric contraction — Development of muscular tension without a change of muscular length.

Isotonic contraction — The shortening of a muscle as it develops tension.

Joint flexibility — Same as flexibility.

Kilocalorie — A thousand calories.

Kilogram — A metric unit of weight equal to 1000 grams and to 2.2 pounds.

Lactic acid — A chemical formed during the incomplete chemical breakdown of carbohydrate that causes muscular fatigue.

Lean body weight — Same as fat-free weight.

Maximal oxygen consumption — The maximal rate at which the muscles can consume oxygen in one minute. Also called maximal aerobic power.

Maximum heart rate reserve — Difference between resting and maximum heart rate.

Mental fitness — Same as emotional fitness.

Metabolism — The various series of chemical reactions involved in energy production that take place within the human body.

Minerals — Food nutrients found in trace amounts in the body and important to proper bodily function, for example, calcium, phosphorus, potassium, sodium, iron, and iodine.

Mitochondria — Subcellular structures found in cells where aerobic metabolism takes place.

Motor fitness — The abilities related to physical skills.

Motor nerve — A nerve cell supplying a muscle and which, when stimulated, causes muscular contraction.

Motor unit — A motor nerve and all the muscle fibers it supplies.

Muscular endurance — The length of time a muscle or muscle group can continue to exert force without fatiguing.

Muscular fitness — Concerned with muscular strength, muscular endurance, and joint flexibility.

Muscular strength — Same as strength.

Myofibril — That part of a muscle fiber containing two protein filaments, actin and myosin.

Myosin — A protein contained in muscle and involved in muscular contraction.

Neuromuscular — Pertaining to the nervous and muscular systems.

Neuromuscular junction — The joining of a muscle and its nerve.

Nutritional fitness — Proper selection of foods with regard to their nutrient and caloric values as well as proper eating habits.

Nutrition — The science of food as it relates to optimal health and performance.

Obese — Overfat.

Obesity — The above-average amount of fat contained in the body.

Overload — To exercise a muscle or muscle group against resistances that exceed those normally encountered.

Oxygen transport system — The cardiorespiratory system or the heart-lung system.

Perimysium — The connective tissue that surrounds a group or bundle of muscle fibers.

Progressive resistance — Overloading a muscle or muscle group throughout the duration of a weight resistance program.

Pulmonary ventilation — The movement of air into and out of the lungs.

Pulse rate — Heart rate.

Protein — A basic foodstuff containing amino acids.

Quality of life — An overall positive feeling and enthusiasm for life.

Sarcolemma — The cell membrane of a muscle fiber.

Saturated fat — Animal fats and fats found in eggs and dairy products and that contribute toward atherosclerosis.

Sensory nerve — A nerve that conveys information from an organ to the central nervous system.

Skinfold — A pinch of skin and subcutaneous fat from which total body fat may be estimated.

Skinfold caliper — An instrument used to measure the thickness of a skinfold.

Slow-twitch fiber — A muscle fiber characterized by slow contraction time, high aerobic metabolism, and low anaerobic metabolism.

Spot reducing — A myth that fat can selectively be lost from one body area through exercise.

Strength — The capacity of a muscle or muscle group to develop force during contraction.

Stroke volume — The amount of blood pumped by the heart with each beat.

Subcutaneous fat — Fat deposits and storage under the skin.

Target heart rate — A predetermined heart rate to be obtained during exercise training.

Thrombus — A blood clot.

Tissue-capillary membrane — The site at which gas exchanges take place between blood and tissue.

Underload — To work a muscle or muscle group at a resistance or load that is normally encountered.

Unsaturated fat — Fats found in vegetable oils and that do not contribute toward atherosclerosis.

Venous blood — Blood low in oxygen and high in carbon dioxide.

Ventilation — Same as pulmonary ventilation.

Vitamins — Food nutrients in the presence of which important metabolic reactions occur.

Selected References and Readings

Allsen, P., Harrison, J., and Vance, B.: *Fitness for Life,* Dubuque, Iowa, Wm. C. Brown, 1980.

Corbin, C., and Lindsey, R.: *Fitness for Life,* Glenview, Ill., Scott, Foresman and Company, 1979.

Dusek, D. E.: *Thin and Fit: Your Personal Lifestyle,* Belmont, Cal., Wadsworth Publishing Company, 1982.

Falls, H. B., Baylor, A. M., and Dishman, R. K.: *Essentials of Fitness,* Philadelphia, Saunders College Publishing, 1980.

Fisher, A. G., and Conlee, R.: *The Complete Book of Physical Fitness,* Provo, Utah, Brigham Young University Press, 1979.

Fox, E. L., and Mathews, D. K.: *Interval Training,* Philadelphia, W. B. Saunders Company, 1974.

Fox, E. L., and Mathews, D. K.: *The Physiological Basis of Physical Education and Athletics,* 3rd ed., Philadelphia, Saunders College Publishing, 1981.

Fox, E. L., Mathews, D. K., and Bairstow, J. N.: *I.T.: Interval Training for Lifetime Fitness,* New York, Dial Press, 1980.

Fox. E. L.: *Sports Physiology,* Philadelphia, Saunders College Publishing, 1979.

Getchell, B.: *Physical Fitness: A Way of Life,* 2nd ed., New York, John Wiley and Sons, 1979.

Hockey, R. V.: *Physical Fitness,* 3rd ed., St. Louis, C. V. Mosby Company, 1978.

Katch, F. I., and McArdle, W. D.: *Nutrition, Weight Control and Exercise,* Boston, Houghton Mifflin, 1977.

Melograno, V., and Klinzing, J.: *An Orientation to Total Fitness,* Dubuque, Iowa, Kendall/Hunt Publishing Company, 1974.

Miller, D. K., and Allen, T. E.: *Fitness: A Lifetime Commitment,* Minneapolis, Burgess Publishing Company, 1979.

Pollock, M. L., Wilmore, J. H., and Fox, S. M.: *Health and Fitness Through Physical Activity,* New York, John Wiley and Sons, 1978.

Smith, N. J.: *Food for Sport,* Palo Alto, Cal., Bull Publishing Company, 1976.

Stokes, R., Moore, A. C., Moore, C., and Williams, C.: *Fitness: The New Wave,* Winston-Salem, Hunter Publishing Company, 1981.

INDEX

A

Actin, 25
Adenosine triphosphate (*see* ATP)
Adipocytes, 79
Adipose tissue, 79
Aerobic, definition of, 16
Aerobic fitness (*see* endurance fitness)
Aerobic metabolism, 16, 18
Alveolar-capillary membrane, 21
Alveoli, 21
Amenorrhea, 80
Amino acids, 69
Anaerobic, definition of, 16
Anaerobic metabolism, 16, 18
Aneurysm, 12
Aphasia, 12
Arm curl, 57, 64
Atherosclerosis, 2
ATP, 17

B

Back hyperextension, 58
Barbells,
    compared with Nautilus and Universal, 64
    exercises for, 66
Basic food groups, 74
Bench press, 57
Bench Step Test, 103
Bent-arm pullover, 56
Bent-knee sit-ups, 63
    as test for muscular endurance, 114
Bent-over rowing, 60
Blood cholesterol levels, 6
Blood clot, endurance training and, 31
Blood flow, 22
Blood pressure, 7
Body composition,
    evaluation of, 117-124
    ideal body weight and, 122
    muscular fitness programs and, 48
    skinfold thickness and, 119

Body composition (*Continued*)
    underwater weighing and, 119
    weight control and, 79
Body fat, loss of, 94-97
Body weight, ideal, 122
Body weight control, 79-99
    adipocytes and, 79
    amenorrhea and, 80
    body composition and, 79
    body fat and, 79
    caloric deficit and, 95
    caloric expenditure and, 83
    caloric intake and, 83
    gaining muscle mass (lean body weight)
        and, 97-99
    height-weight table and, 82
    lean body weight and, 80
    losing body fat and, 94
    obesity and, 80
    questions and answers about, 133
    spot reducing and, 97
    water loss vs. fat loss and, 96

C

Caloric deficit, 95
Caloric expenditure, estimation of, 83-85
Caloric intake, estimation of, 83
Caloric needs, 72
Caloric values of foods, table of, 86-94
Carbohydrates,
    anaerobic metabolism and, 18
    as food nutrient, 69
    as pregame meal, 77
Cardiac dysrhythmias, endurance training
    and, 31
Cardiac output, 22
Cardiorespiratory fitness, definition of, 13
Cardiorespiratory fitness programs, 29-45
    (*see also* endurance fitness programs)
Cardiorespiratory system,
    alveolar-capillary membrane and, 21
    alveoli and, 21